praise for whole mama Yoga

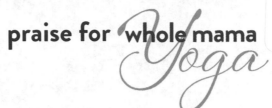

"Alexandra and Lauren are gifted teachers—I know this from working alongside them for over twenty years, during which both of them became mothers. In this compassionate, friendly book, they guide you toward greater connection with yourself, your child, and your community. This connection is yoga. Best of all, *Whole Mama Yoga* meets you where you are—no yoga experience needed—and points you toward practices and philosophy that will help you feel held and nurtured even as you work to hold and nurture your child. *Whole Mama Yoga* is an invaluable guide for every state of the journey, from preconception through parenting. It will make the perfect gift for your friends and family as they embark on the road to parenthood."

—**Sage Rountree, PhD, E-RYT 500,** co-owner of Carolina Yoga Company, author of *Everyday Yoga*

"*Whole Mama Yoga* does a great job exploring how yoga practice can support parents along the spectrum of preconception, pregnancy, and postpartum. It presents a welcome balance between evidence-based information from experts and deeply personal stories. This book offers a refreshingly down to earth and supportive take on the many benefits of yoga for the parent-to-be and new parent, while putting to rest some common misconceptions about yoga during pregnancy. Highly recommend!"

—**Libby Hinsley, PT, DPT, C-IAYT, E-RYT 500, YACEP,** author of *Yoga for Bendy People*

"No matter where you are on your journey into motherhood, Alexandra and Lauren are the wise and compassionate companions you need to navigate this most precious and auspicious time in your life. Through practical advice, meditations, movements, and moments of reflection, *Whole Mama Yoga* gives you everything you need to remember and deeply connect with your innate ability to mindfully and lovingly enter into parenthood. *Whole Mama Yoga* should be an integral part of every mama's birthing (and parenting) team."

—**Linda Sparrowe,** author of *YogaMama: The Practitioner's Guide to Prenatal Yoga*

whole mama Yoga

Meditation, Mantra, and Movement for Pregnancy and Beyond

Alexandra DeSiato and Lauren Sacks

Health Communications, Inc.
Boca Raton, Florida

www.hcibooks.com

Library of Congress Cataloging-in-Publication Data

DeSiato, Alexandra, author. | Sacks, Lauren, author.

Whole mama yoga: your journey from preconception through pregnancy,
    birth & parenthood / by Alexandra DeSiato and Lauren Sacks.
Boca Raton, FL: Health Communications, Inc., [2023] |
    Includes bibliographical references.
LCCN 2023006618 (print) | LCCN 2023006619 (ebook) |
ISBN 9780757324666 (paperback) | ISBN 0757324665 (paperback) |
ISBN 9780757324673 (epub) | ISBN 0757324673 (epub)
LCSH: Exercise for pregnant women. | Physical fitness for pregnant women. | Yoga—Popular works. |
    Pregnant women--Health and hygiene--Popular works. | Mothers--Health and hygiene--Popular works.
LCC RG558.7 .D47 2023 (print) | LCC RG558.7 (ebook) | DDC
    618.2/44--dc23/eng/20230428

LC record available at https://lccn.loc.gov/2023006618
LC ebook record available at https://lccn.loc.gov/2023006619

HCI, its logos, and marks are trademarks of Health Communications, Inc.

Publisher: Health Communications, Inc.
        301 Crawford Boulevard, Suite 200
        Boca Raton, FL 33432–3762

Cover, interior design, and formatting by Larissa Hise Henoch

contents

foreword

by Mary Ochsner

Life as I knew it would flip upside down. I held the positive pregnancy test in my hands, shaking in disbelief that it was actually happening. I knew this was the beginning of an exciting new chapter of life; yet I felt terrified and nervous, all at the same time. I took a slow deep breath, savoring the moment and trusting that I'd be supported and guided through this new experience.

As an avid yogi and yoga teacher, I knew my yoga practice would be shifting in the months to come. I started to do some research on prenatal yoga and was shocked at the amount of vague, fear-inducing, and contradicting information out there. As a yoga teacher to thousands of yogis around the world, I thought I would feel more confident in practicing yoga while I was pregnant. But I didn't. I felt scared, unsure of what to do, and not wanting to do anything to injure myself or harm my baby. I knew if I felt this scared around practicing yoga while pregnant, there had to be many others feeling the same.

Yoga can be one of the most beneficial practices to do while you're pregnant. It guides you to love and support your ever-changing body. It slows down your busy mind, connects you deeper within, and teaches you how to breathe deep in the most challenging moments. It nourishes your soul and prepares you for the most incredible life transformation. Unfortunately, many pregnant people feel at a loss on how to get started, how to practice safely, and how to properly incorporate this practice into their pregnancy journey. Even as a yoga teacher with years of experience, I still felt this way.

When I learned about the Whole Mama Yoga Prenatal and Postnatal Teacher Training, I signed up immediately. Not only did I crave the support myself, but I wanted to support my students who desired to incorporate yoga into their pregnancy experience. I had previously connected with Alexandra because of *Teaching Yoga Beyond the Poses,* and knew I wanted her mentorship as I started my journey as a prenatal yoga teacher.

Learning from both Alexandra and Lauren has been one of the greatest blessings on my yoga journey. With their guidance I went from feeling fearful about practicing yoga while pregnant to feeling fully empowered in my body and practice. They taught me how to listen to my motherly instincts, connect to the new sensations in my body, feel confident and strong not only on my mat, but off my mat as well. I learned to trust my body through this process, and I know this brought more peace and ease to not only my pregnancy, but also my labor and delivery, and my transition into motherhood.

Whole Mama Yoga: Meditation, Mantra, and Movement for Pregnancy and Beyond is the resource I wish I had when I first became pregnant. It's exhausting to sift through the noise out there about what to do or not do while you're pregnant. What I love about this book is it takes you deeper than just practicing yoga poses: You get the full yoga experience. This book invites you to intentionally move your body, turn inward, slow down, breathe deeply, reflect on your experience, connect with others, and lean on the wisdom from those already on their motherhood journey.

What I love about this book is it takes you deeper than just practicing yoga poses: You get the full yoga experience.

As you make your way through this book, you'll notice a common theme that I learned from Alexandra and Lauren, which is: *You are your own best teacher.* Read that again. This wise advice doesn't only apply to prenatal yoga, pregnancy, or stepping into parenthood. This is a lesson that will change your entire life. When you can step into that power, when you trust your own inner voice and live with confidence, your whole world will change. This book gives you the wisdom to harness that deep knowing we all have within.

Pregnancy and parenthood have been the most rewarding, yet challenging, experiences of my life. This book will give you the tools you need to flow through these tough moments with grace. Instead of being reactive, you'll learn to pause and take a deep breath. As your body changes week by week, you'll learn how to move in ways that ease your aches and pains. If you're feeling stressed, overwhelmed, or anxious, you'll have an abundance of meditations, affirmations, and mantras to bring you back to your center. In tense moments, you'll have breathing techniques you can practice to calm your mind and nervous system. There is space for reflection, to process the intense emotions you may be experiencing and advice from others who have been through what you're going through and can offer guidance from their experience. There are times when we do feel so isolated, yet this book is our connection to that community of others to remind us we are not alone.

Let this book be your trusted guide on the most incredible, life-changing journey of pregnancy and parenthood. The skills and mindset shifts you'll learn in these pages are invaluable during this chapter of life. Having Alexandra and Lauren's guidance at your fingertips will be the breath of fresh air that you need to ride the waves that come your way—just as I did when I first found out I was becoming a mother.

Take a deep breath. Trust that, with the knowledge you hold in your hands and your internal instincts, you'll be guided and supported every step of the way. You've got this!

—Mary Ochsner

introduction

Welcome to the journey of motherhood and parenthood. We're so glad you've found our book along this path! We've written it as mothers, yoga practitioners and teachers, and fellow travelers on this journey. This book is informed by all those experiences, and it includes reflections and wisdom from others also on this journey. One of our intentions for this book is that it be yours for the duration of this trip, and you may use it at all stations. Yoga's own path and practice is lifelong, and we have both leaned heavily on yoga's tools—particularly those we have discovered during our own practice—to provide us support. We offer thoughts and guidance on preconception, being pregnant, arriving into motherhood, navigating the postpartum period, and active parenting.

Throughout the book, you'll find sections titled MOVE that offer yoga poses and sequences for each part of the journey. We offer REFLECT as a way to give you options for meditations that may offer a balm for your soul. You'll also find short mantras that can be repeated or chanted to help you feel grounded and present, or even just as opportunities for self-reflection. BREATHE offers helpful breathing techniques and *pranayama* practices. In WISDOM, you'll find sweet yoga tidbits, philosophy, and lessons from Ayurveda as they apply to motherhood and parenthood. We've also pulled wisdom from our friends in the fields of perinatal and maternal wellness, mental health, Ayurveda, physical therapy, sleep, and more. RELATE is a chance for you to hear from other moms and parents who have also used yoga poses and philosophy along the way.

Almost immediately when you begin trying to get pregnant, you are bombarded with advice. You may get advice from friends or family about ovulation, patience, or even the best positions to foster conception (!). This advising will continue once you are pregnant. You'll hear advice on what not to eat or drink (and what to eat and drink), when you should reveal your pregnancy, how to decide your baby's name, what laboring choices you should make, what bassinet to buy (but why does it matter because "You'll never sleep again!"), and on and on and on. When your child arrives, you'll be advised on how to best care for them, how to parent effectively, how to love your child or not spoil your baby, and the best way to burp, swaddle, or bathe your little one. There is no end to the inundation of advice, and we've both felt the pressure that advice can exert. Even for people who have long trusted their internal compass, this completely new, and sometimes confusing, experience seems to require (and provoke) *so much* external input. Because we know first-hand (and second) how overwhelming and confusing well-intentioned advice can be to expecting and new parents, our only advice to you is to listen to yourself. And we hope you'll find some wisdom in this book.

There is no end to the inundation of advice, and we've both felt the pressure that advice can exert.

An important intention for us in writing this book is to help you come back to yourself. You know your body best, and you will know your baby best. Your intuition is a force that can be trusted, and your sense of how best to care for and love yourself and your child should always be the loudest voice you heed. In yoga, this sense of right-seeing is called *vidya*. Listening to yourself does not mean letting ego (*asmita*) guide you. It means that because you practice self-awareness, you trust yourself. We trust you. That's why you'll find that this book is about suggestions from yoga that may be useful to you on this path, and it has less to do with what *not* to do: you know already, or if you don't, you'll seek that out from trusted experts you have wisely chosen.

Our expertise is yoga. In this book, you'll find sequences that are safe for you to do wherever you are on the path. You'll find suggestions for poses and movements to avoid and suggestions for poses and movements that might help with the ills of pregnancy or the stressors of parenthood. You'll find breath practices that can help you feel grounded, less anxious, or more energized. You'll find movement, breath, and other tools of yoga that have guided our own motherhood paths.

In tandem with this book, we have a website: *wholemamayoga.com*. On this website, you'll find videos of many of the sequences from this book, examples of breath practices, and chants and mantras we offer here. We want yoga to be accessible to you through your motherhood journey, and we hope this helps increase that accessibility.

It's likely that you chose this book because you already practice yoga, either casually or with dedication. There's something about the path of yoga—maybe the marriage of movement science with magical transformation—that speaks to you on an intrinsic, spiritual level. But if you chose this book thinking *Huh, maybe I should start yoga now!* well, good news: You're right. This is the perfect time to start yoga.

This is the perfect time to start yoga because the very definition of yoga is *union* or *yoke*. Your path to motherhood or parenthood is a yoking: You're yoking part of your soul to another being. In the next few months and years, you'll be paying attention to signs of your ovulation, your growing baby, your shifting body, and yourself in ways you may never have previously. This newly paid attention isn't narcissism: It's mindfulness and presence. Renowned Buddhist monk Thich Nhat Hanh says, "Every act is a rite." Every breath you take is an experience of mindfulness; every dish you wash is meditation. As you start to notice your body now, you are dropping into mindful, present awareness.

This is the perfect time to start yoga because data supports the physical practice of yoga as a healthy and helpful movement practice during pregnancy and the postpartum period. From The American College of Obstetricians and Gynecologists (ACOG) website (www.acog.org): "Yoga reduces stress, improves flexibility, and encourages stretching and focused breathing." In her book *Expecting Better*, economist and data scientist Emily Oster notes that according to some small studies, "labor was two and a half hours shorter" for the group of participants that did yoga. She concludes, "Prenatal yoga is definitely worth trying . . . If nothing else, perhaps you will improve your self-actualization."

Oster may have been being tongue-in-cheek with that "self-actualization" bit, but as we've already noted, the path of yoga is one of presence and mindfulness. It makes sense that as you embark on this journey, you seek ways not just to connect with your body (and eventual baby), not just to move safely and stay strong, but that you also seek ways to know yourself more deeply and fully.

Yoga has been a guiding force for us both as moms. The philosophy of yoga has helped us in our parenting choices and helped us consider our relationship with ourselves. The breath practices of yoga have given us an anchor for our attention, and a tool for calming our minds (or sometimes energizing our bodies). The physical poses and movements of yoga—the *asanas*—have given us a chance to have tactile, tangible relationships with our own bodies as they've changed through motherhood. Yoga asana has sometimes given us a chance to find space from our motherhood roles (on our mats or in a class or in a retreat). Sometimes we move our bodies in yoga as a tool of coping with discomfort, whether that be physical or existential. Often, we move our bodies in yoga because it's pleasurable, joyful, and grounding, enabling us to connect to our spiritual selves through our physical selves.

The philosophy of yoga has helped us in our parenting choices and helped us consider our relationship with ourselves.

Whatever reason you chose this book, we're so glad you're here! Motherhood and parenthood will change you: physically, spiritually, and emotionally. Yoga serves as a light along the way.

Part One

preconception

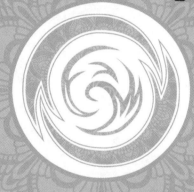

Chapter One

making space for baby

Woo-hoo! You have taken the first big step in your parenting journey: deciding to start trying to grow or build your family. Making this decision requires a great deal of courage and self-awareness. It's an exciting time that may lend itself to heart-opening, hopefulness, and a stronger sense of your intuitive self. This is also the time to cultivate patience as the timeline unfolds at its own pace.

Growth and change don't happen without obstacles or strife. Fortunately, yoga meets you where you are—we have both cried during practice, heavy with grief, and we've also felt enormous weight lift as a result. Yoga allows us to bear witness and more deeply observe our inner selves. By creating this deeper connection within, it becomes a little easier to quiet external noise and tap into what makes most sense in our own lives.

In yoga philosophy, the concept of *tapas* means something akin to fiery devotion to your practice; your internal heat; your sense of self-discipline, drive, passion, and vigor. Becoming a parent requires tapas. This huge life shift takes tremendous courage—and having courage doesn't mean you're acting without fear. It just means you're moving forward in the face of fear, taking action regardless.

Along with courage, though, the move from person to parent requires a sort of heart-opening, a shifting of priorities, a space-making. Self-compassion—*karuna* in yoga philosophy—is necessary. Deciding to become a parent means that you're opening a new part of yourself and your life. In all

7

this shifting, you might recognize a desire to mourn or grieve the life you are moving away from or leaving behind. Looking at all this change through the lens of karuna can help you be kinder and gentler to yourself in this process. All aspects of yoga—the physical practice, the breathwork, the philosophy, and the mantra and meditation will be useful for stabilizing and grounding during tumultuous times of transformation and change, like this one. Although the transformation into motherhood is huge, inhabiting a body, especially one with female sex hormones, is to constantly be subject to transition—something you already know from lived experience. The practice of yoga is a practice well-suited to women and birthing people because it has balance at its core: yoga seeks an alignment of opposing energies in order to find a place, a home, in the middle.

The practice of yoga is a practice well-suited to women and birthing people because it has balance at its core.

One other thing we'd like to address here: We hope you're beginning this new exploration of courage and heart-opening from a place of excitement, but we want to honor any fear, sadness, or trauma you may also be experiencing. Maybe you've had miscarriages, or you chose to terminate an earlier pregnancy. Maybe grief and longing are part of this experience. Maybe you have a family history of concerning illnesses or a childhood that is painful and brings to mind fear of being a mother or parent yourself. If these harder emotions are also part of this awakening into parenthood, a trusted therapist can help you process these experiences, not so that you arrive in a field of rainbows and abundant bliss, but to understand your own self, and in that understanding, find wisdom to move forward.

So here you go, forward into the unknown, trusting that the path ahead—though shrouded in mystery and unfolding at its own pace—is the right one for you.

MOVE
yoga for patience

Once you've made the decision to get pregnant, waiting becomes nuanced and may feel difficult. Waiting is a huge part of parenting, too (minutes never go by as slowly as when waiting for a toddler to climb into their own car seat), so practicing this skill now grows your capacity for the depth of patience required throughout parenthood. Sitting in stillness can feel impossible, and movement of your physical body can be helpful in quieting your mind. You can complete the movements in this sequence as many times as you'd like, or you can add in other flowing poses to create more dynamic movement before you come to stillness.

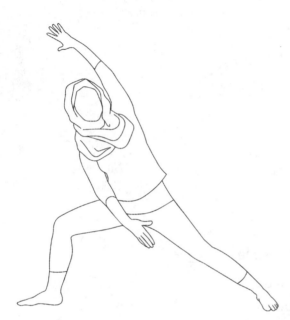

Side angle pose variation

Take a wide stance on your mat, with your right foot pointing to the front of your mat and your left foot angled toward the right long edge of your mat. Bend your right knee and pause for a moment in Warrior 2, with your arms shoulder height, parallel to the floor. Stretch your left arm alongside your ear while simultaneously sweeping your right arm to hover above the top of your left thigh.

Reverse warrior variation

From side angle pose, lean your torso toward the back of your mat. Keep the position of your legs and your stance the same and sweep your left arm back and then forward to hover next to the inside of your front thigh. At the same time, sweep your right arm back and up to extend alongside your right ear.

Flow between these two poses several times, pausing to rest with a forearm on your thigh or by straightening both legs.

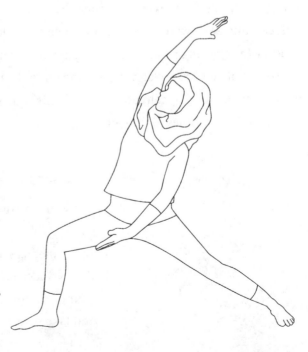

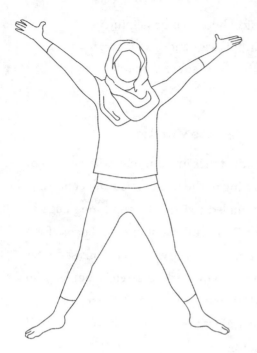

Malasana **flow start**

To start this flowing *malasana*, or squat flow, step in from your wide stance so that your feet are shoulder-distance apart. Turn your feet outward. Take a deep breath in and sweep your arms up and overhead.

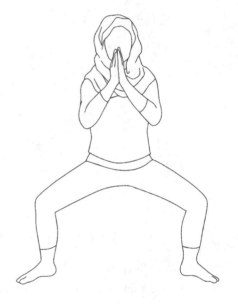

Malasana **flow middle**

Bring your hands together overhead and then allow your palms to trace a line downward as you begin to bend your knees and enter into a squatting position, exhaling as you move. You can choose to hold a deep squat here, moving on to the next pose in the sequence, or you can move through this squat-to-stand flow several more times to find an energizing flow.

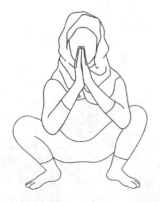

Malasana **hold**

Settle into a squatting position, taking your knees as wide as is comfortable for your body. If you're able to bring your elbows to your inner legs, do so, and press your upper arms into your inner thighs and your inner thighs back into your upper arms. Press your palms together to help with this engagement. Close your eyes and take several full breaths here.

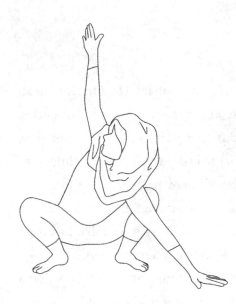

Malasana twist

Maintaining the position of your feet and legs, move your left hand to the outside of your left shin and place it on the ground. Bring your right hand to the top of your right knee and twist right. You can also stretch your arm skyward. Hold this twist for several breaths before switching to twist to the other side.

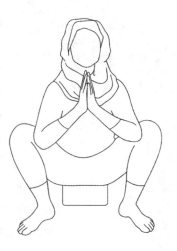

Malasana meditation

If you're comfortable remaining in this squatting position, stay here for a few more breaths, or bring a bolster, pillow, or block(s) under you instead. Take a few rounds of breaths, imagining a light filling up the space of your belly and pelvis. The light can begin as a small flame, with each inhalation encouraging the light to expand and grow.

Repeat this sequence again, placing your right foot at the top of your mat for the first two poses.

REFLECT
chanting to remove obstacles

In the Hindu faith, the god Ganesha is part man, part elephant. He is the lord of all living things, and the bringer of good luck. He's also known as the remover of obstacles. When starting important endeavors, devout Hindus often seek Ganesha's blessings. A *ganpati* mantra, or mantra to Ganesha, is a reminder to bring all his good qualities into us. When we chant this, we might do it in the spirit of removing negativities to ensure our new venture, journey, or path is one of success. As you start on the road to creating a child, this mantra can serve as a powerful way to feel like this is an auspicious beginning and you are protected in the endeavor.

The ganpati mantra, or mantra to Ganesha, is a reminder to bring all his good qualities into us.

Find a comfortable seat—a chair is just fine, or you might sit on a cushion or the floor. Chanting a mantra can feel strange to Westerners if you're new to this practice. Chanting is like singing in that it creates sounds and vibrations that can feel soothing. You don't have to practice Hinduism or even have religious faith to find peace in words that evoke a sense of safety on your chosen path. (But if you do practice a faith tradition, you might already have powerful mantras or affirmations that speak to you from the liturgy and texts of your faith.)

Once you find a comfortable seat, turn your attention to your breath, allowing it to slow and deepen. You might even take a few open-mouth sighs. Then, start to chant:

Om Gam Ganapataye Namaha

The internet abounds with versions of this chant if you're curious about the typical rhythm of it or aren't certain of pronunciation. (And of course, our companion website also includes this chant, so you can hear it directly from us.)

You might chant quietly at first, but as you feel comfortable with the words and phrasing, let your voice grow louder. There is no hard and fast rule for how many times you can chant this, but often in Sanskrit (the sacred language of yoga) mantras are chanted in multiples of nine, up to one hundred eight times.

pranayama and prana

If you've heard the term *pranayama* in yoga class, you probably know it means breath practice or retention. But the root of that word is the word *prana*. The definition of this Sanskrit term can be tricky to pin down in English. It means life force, certainly. And, too, it means breath. The idea of prana is that it exists everywhere: in us and around us. One commonly used analogy is to imagine a jar of water floating in an ocean. The water in the jar is prana contained (as it becomes contained in each of us!) and the water in the ocean is also prana. It is the stuff of life. In yoga philosophy, we use pranayama, or breathing techniques, to guide prana through our bodies—into them and out of them—clearing a path. That's why breathing practices in yoga have a sacredness to them. We aren't just breathing; we're using our breath to stir our very life force and connect with the energy all around us. In engaging in breath practices, you are calling more life force into your body. But here's the part of yoga that we love so much: You don't have to believe in the unseen, unproven parts of it to derive the benefit of the tools and practice.

As a mom-or-parent-to-be, whether you are interested in the concept of prana or not doesn't really matter. Science tells us that breath practices work. They work to lessen anxiety by signaling to your nervous system to calm down. When you breathe more slowly and more deeply, you offer tranquility to your mind, which is of benefit to anyone, anytime—and maybe especially to you right now. As humans in the world as it currently is, we spend a lot of time in our *sympathetic* nervous system—helpful when we need to run quickly away from something, not as helpful when we need to slow down and allow our body's natural rhythms and processes to take over. Intentional focus on the breath provides a gateway to the *parasympathetic* nervous system, giving our bodies and brains the signal that all is well and that we are safe.

MOVE
yoga for heart-opening

Vulnerability is hard. To attempt to conceive opens you up to a vast array of emotions—from disappointment to elation. We live in a world that promotes walling ourselves off, in both a physical and emotional sense. Giving birth to a child, and raising that child, however, requires us to do quite the opposite. Children break our hearts wide *open*. In preparation for embracing that vulnerability of both trying to conceive and then of becoming a parent, practice this exposed-heart sequence that gives you a chance to connect to yourself through movement and allows you to start to open yourself to the great possibility of parenthood. Two blocks (or something similar) are helpful for the following poses.

Supine heart-opening with blocks

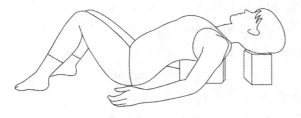

Place your blocks toward the back of your mat. One block should be placed under your head at the middle height, and the other block should be placed in between your shoulder blades and in line with your spine. This block can be placed at any height; the higher you go, the more intense the chest opening. Lie down with the blocks supporting your head and back and extend your arms out to either side. Place your feet on the floor, outer hip distance apart, and rest your inner knees together. Remain here for three to five minutes, relaxing your arms toward the floor.

Sukhasana with hands behind

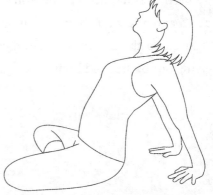

Come up to a cross-legged (*sukhasana*) seated position, and place your hands about a foot behind you, with your fingertips facing toward your body. On an inhalation, rise up to your fingertips and begin to bend your elbows, lifting your gaze slightly. As you breathe out, relax your belly and bring your spine back to a neutral position. Repeat this movement a few times.

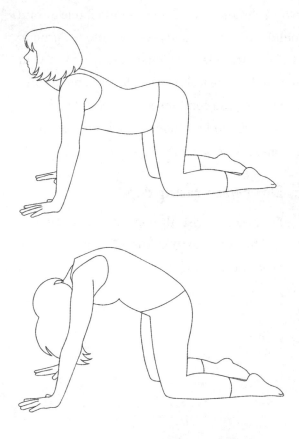

Cat and cow

Come up to your hands and knees, with your hands under your shoulders and your knees under your hips. Press your hands actively into the ground. As you begin your inhale, slowly lift your tailbone, drop your belly, lift your chest and, finally, your gaze. As you release your breath, begin to round your back and scoop your tailbone under. Repeat this several times, allowing the movement of your body to follow the rhythm of your breath.

Cobra explorations

From hands and knees, lower to your belly and bring your hands in line with your chest. For the first cobra pose, focus on pressing the tops of your feet into the floor and keeping your low back long. Press your hands very gently into the floor and lift your head and shoulders. Lower back to your belly. For the second round, press your hands more actively into the floor and begin to lift your chest off the floor, as you continue to press into the tops of your feet.

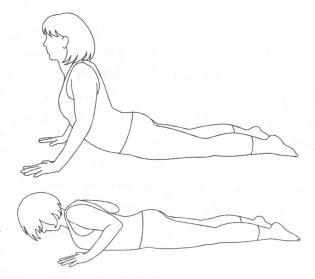

Maintain length in your lower back by engaging your low belly and lengthening your tailbone toward your heels. Lower back to the ground. For the final round, press your hands actively into the ground and lift your chest fully off the ground. (Do this only if you are able to maintain the length in your lower back. If you feel discomfort there, or if the entirety of the pose feels like it is focused on the area of the low back, come back to one of the previous variations.) As you continue to press your hands into the ground, imagine pulling your hands back toward your lower body without actually moving them. After a couple of breaths here, lower back to the ground and rest for a moment.

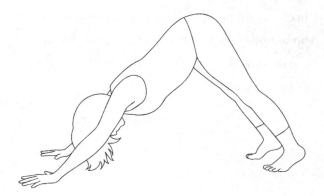

Downward-facing dog

From cobra, rise through hands and knees and lift your hips and knees as you come into downward-facing dog.

Low lunge

From downward-facing dog, stretch your right leg high into the air. Swing your right foot forward and place your foot in between your hands at the top of your mat. (If this is difficult, you can always lower the back knee and scoot your right foot forward or use your hand to help place your foot.) Lower your back knee and bring both hands to your front thigh. Create a scissoring action in your hips, energetically drawing your back hip forward and your front hip backward. Your hands can remain on your front leg or you may stretch them alongside your ears. As with other backbends, focus on opening the chest and upper back while maintaining a sense of stability in the low back.

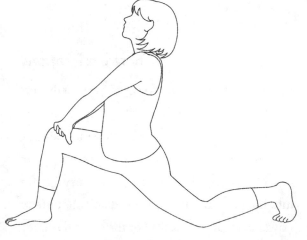

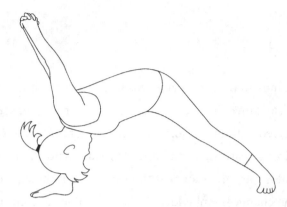

Humble warrior

From low lunge, lower the sole of your back foot, angling it at a 45-degree angle facing the front of your mat. Rise up to standing and interlace your fingers at the small of your back. Keeping your fingers interlaced, bring your torso to the inside of your front leg, allowing the crown of your head to drop toward the floor.

Return to downward-facing dog and repeat the previous two poses on the second side.

Puppy pose

From warrior, place both hands on the ground and step your feet back to downward-facing dog. Lower your knees and walk your hands forward until your forehead is on the ground. Keep your hips stacked over your knees. Spread your hands as wide or wider than your mat, and stretch your arms out long, softening the space between your shoulder blades toward your mat.

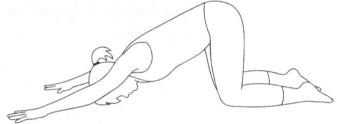

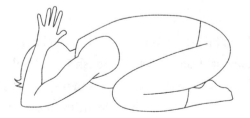

Child's pose with shoulder release

From puppy pose, lower your hips back toward your heels and allow them to rest there. Walk your arms back to a comfortable position. If you'd like more of a stretch in your shoulders, bend your elbows and bring your hands into a prayer position at the back of your head.

REFLECT
affirmations for staying grounded

Language is a powerful tool, not only in the way that words impact others, but also in the way that the words we speak (or think) to ourselves affect our own way of seeing and being in the world. When faced with an important decision, remind yourself about the flow of life, its always-shifting seasons, and the fundamental truth that the only constant is change. In yoga philosophy, the idea that the central, natural state of the universe is constant evolution and change is embedded in the cosmological concept of *parinamavada*. In the face of all that constant change, we can use the tools of yoga to stay grounded.

We like to use affirmations (repeated phrases, in your mind or spoken out loud) or mantras (chanted phrases, which we'll look at more in future chapters) as one way to reflect on this shifting sense of life. Here are a few helpful ones:

The only constant is change.
I let go and flow on the path.
I don't have to be in charge.
This is life, unfolding.
Hold on. Let go.

BREATHE
build heat and stoke your fire

An empowering breath practice, *kapalabhati* breathing is a good way to feel a little more alive and connected to yourself. Kapalabhati translates from Sanskrit as "skull-shining breath," but don't let that translation intimidate you. Think of it as a way to get a little more clearheaded. In traditional yogic thinking, this breath is cleansing and rejuvenating. Some breath practices can make us feel as if we're breathing out the tiredness and sluggishness and heaviness, and this is definitely one of them!

During this breath, your inhalation is mellow and more relaxed, but your exhalation is strong and forceful. When you first begin this breath, start slowly. We remember feeling like we were running out of breath the first few times we practiced this, so be sure you are also inhaling, even though the focus is on the powerful exhale. Once you become more accustomed to the breath practice, your inhalation is much less conscious—your exhalation naturally creates space for the intake of your breath.

To start, sit tall, your hands resting on your belly. Inhale through your nose, filling your lungs up mostly but not completely. As you quickly exhale—again through your nose—draw your belly button toward your spine and notice that your belly space moves with a sort of gentle jerk inward. Repeat this cycle, with your abdominals contracting on the exhalations and then softening on the inhalations—ten to twenty times. After that, rest and allow your breathing to return to your normal tempo and pace. If you still feel like you need a little more brightening, try another round of ten to twenty. Repeat until you feel more invigorated and clearheaded.

RELATE
mindfulness on the path

Nancy, a yogi, avid biker, and professional, ponders being on the path of trying to get pregnant.

As I reflect on this time when I'm trying to become pregnant, I reflect on a full range of emotions, from excitement and joy to full-on terror, with fear being my closest companion. After my partner and I decided together to embark on creating a family and received approval from my cardiologist (because of a preexisting heart condition), fear began to creep into my mind with consuming thoughts of *You're thirty-seven years old. You're too old.*

Before taking the steps necessary to pursue my desire further, I was halted by my cardiologist's concern that I could have a gene that could be devastating if passed down. Sitting with that news, taking the necessary tests, and then waiting for the results increased my anxiety and fear. During this time, I held tight to my mindfulness practice. There was nothing I could do, no movement, no medication, no therapy possible, to change me from potentially having a gene that would end my hopes of

My yoga practice gives me confidence and calmness.

pregnancy before that pregnancy even began. The mind has the power to destroy you, but my mindfulness practice helped me alter the story of loss that was building in my head. Staying present meant I could make room for hope. This hope allowed me to move forward with all aspects of my life instead of letting the overwhelming fear destroy everything.

Joy filled me when I was given the green light to start trying to conceive. And since I had already waited months at this point, I thought pregnancy would happen immediately.

Each time I start my period, disappointment and fear overcome me again. I've continued with my mindfulness practice to cope with the emotions. The anxiety has lessened. I've allowed and pushed myself to go to the yoga mat. Sweating on my mat reminds me of rebirthing and the opportunity each month provides for another chance. Just as I could barely do Warrior 1 my first time on the mat, I reassure myself of all I have learned in my yoga practice and that I can learn should I have a child. My yoga practice gives me confidence and calmness for another day and another try.

REFLECT
inhale-exhale meditation

If you have a longer amount of time to reflect, try an inhale-exhale meditation. Start by identifying something you'd like to shake off or let go of. It could be an emotion, a fear, or even a physical sensation. Then, imagine the opposite. For instance, if you're trying to let go of anxiety, you might imagine peace. If you want to move away from anticipation, you might think of patience. Find somewhere comfortable to rest. You could lie down, snuggle into a comfy chair, or sit on the ground, resting your seat on a blanket or bolster. Close your eyes, and start to slow your breath, so that you are breathing with more intention. As you inhale, breathe in the emotion, feeling, or sensation you want to cultivate. As you exhale, breathe its opposite out. You might think: *Inhale patience, exhale anticipation.* Or it might sound more like *Inhale peace, exhale anxiety.* Find the words that make you feel empowered to let go and cultivate the strength you need. Find a rhythm that is slow and steady, and if your mind wanders from your intention, gently come back to this affirmation-meditation, inhaling what you need and breathing out what you don't.

yoga for patience

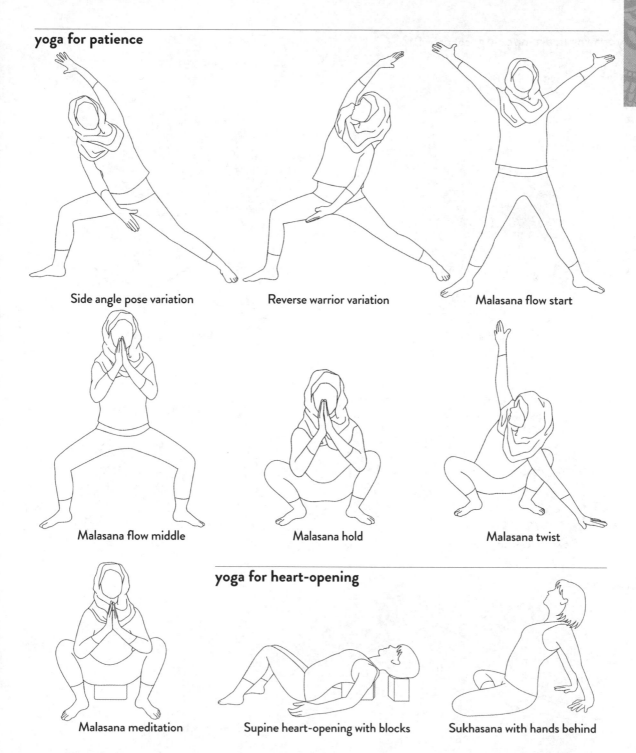

Side angle pose variation   Reverse warrior variation   Malasana flow start

Malasana flow middle   Malasana hold   Malasana twist

Malasana meditation

yoga for heart-opening

Supine heart-opening with blocks   Sukhasana with hands behind

yoga for heart-opening (continued)

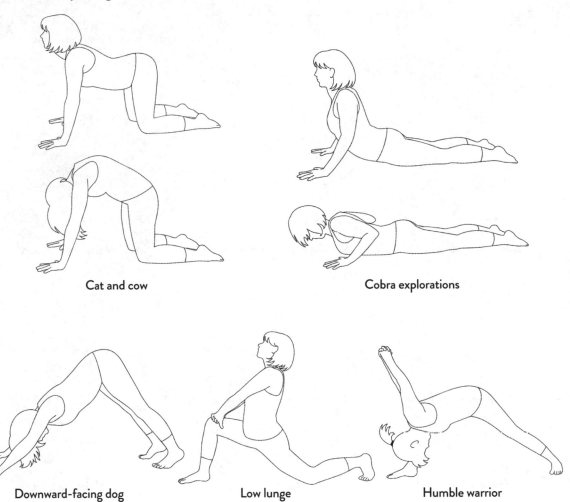

Cat and cow

Cobra explorations

Downward-facing dog

Low lunge

Humble warrior

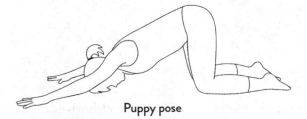

Puppy pose

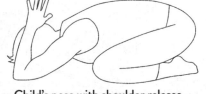

Child's pose with shoulder release

Chapter Two
foundations and fertility

Can yoga help your fertility? One factor in infertility is stress: There is a correlation between higher levels of stress hormones and more challenges getting pregnant. Yoga helps with stress. Stress reduction offers a whole host of health benefits, many of them connected with a better environment for creating life. So yes, we're here to tell you that yoga is a useful complementary alternative therapy when you're on the path of starting a family. Yoga is one (very, very small) piece of the fertility puzzle.

It can be hugely stressful trying to get pregnant. You may have thought it might happen more quickly, or you might not have expected to do more than just have joyful, baby-making sex with your partner. As far as we're aware, no one has found it any easier to let go of stress when told to relax. (Lauren hopes that the anesthesiologist who said that very thing to her prior to her cesarean has also received this feedback.) The fertility journey can feel like a tortuous loop, and sometimes the best we can do is to be present with emotion and sensation in the body, observing and accepting.

While we wish we could offer you a chapter of yoga poses and breathwork that would spontaneously get you pregnant, sometimes bringing a baby into the world takes a circuitous route, and there is not much in your control that can force or make it happen. Instead, yoga offers one means of holding yourself up during times of immense challenge. In the most famous sutra from the *Yoga*

Sutras of Patanjali, we are taught *yoga chitta vritti nirodha*—which means yoga is a path to stilling the fluctuations of the mind. Yoga will not attain anything for you, but it may allow for you to be more fully, exactly where you are.

As much as medical professionals *do* know about fertility, it remains clear that fertility is influenced by a lot of science and a little magic. Our student and friend Dawn shared with us that it was when she connected with her true nature through yoga, meditation, and vivid dreams that she was able to remove her obstacles on the path and become pregnant. In listening to what her inner voice was telling her—in her case, that she needed to fully embrace her bisexuality—she felt she cleared what was blocking her own fertility.

It remains clear that fertility is influenced by a lot of science and a little magic.

On the science side of things, the clearest path is to find a fantastic fertility doctor or clinic if pregnancy isn't happening on the timeline you expected. The general rule is one year of trying for healthy, heterosexual couples over the age of thirty-five, and six months of trying for healthy, heterosexual couples under the age of thirty-five. A fertility expert can guide you through the medical side of fertility, which might include hormone supplementation, medication and injections, intrauterine insemination (IUI), or in vitro fertilization (IVF).

If you're gay, queer, or transgender, your path to parenthood might necessarily take a route that involves support from medical professionals. For the majority of heterosexual couples, conceiving a child is a private endeavor, and medical intervention is a process that for many can feel intrusive and unwanted—however necessary it is to the end goal of parenthood. LGBTQIA+ couples and single individuals often require medical intervention in order to bring a child into the world, and, in addition to the invasion of privacy, the physical and emotional toll of added hormones and procedures, there is often much more of a financial outlay. These challenges of starting a family can add another layer of emotional challenge depending on how supported queer couples and individuals feel throughout the process—both from those closest to them and society at large.

Often the path to having a baby is full of false hope: A late period or a new physical sensation can bring up yearning and expectation that may not come to fruition. In the ups and downs of the journey, your stability comes from within: Your grounding is disconnected from the results of those expectations. We write this knowing that these words may not feel possible to live! How can you not allow hope to lift you up and pain to lower you down? That's not possible, and your emotions will rise and fall, like the waves in the tide. Beneath all that churning and ceaselessness, we invite you to see your wholeness and completeness and calm on a deep, internal level.

RELATE
lauren's fertility story

I was thirty-two when I became pregnant for the first time, the first month of trying to conceive. It was intentional and welcomed and, somehow, still unexpected. I took four at-home pregnancy tests to confirm. It was New Year's Eve and suddenly the world was different.

Events unfolded differently a few years later. At thirty-five, I had crossed over to the so-called "geriatric" side of reproduction and, after trying for six months to conceive on our own, my husband and I sought the guidance of fertility specialists. In order to understand whether intervention was needed, we both had various tests performed. My egg count was "borderline low." Additionally, I am fairly certain the word *wonky* was used to describe the location of my cervix.

Although conception was possible naturally, my physician advised IUI to increase my odds. Even though I was still ovulating, I was prescribed Clomid (a medication designed to increase the hormones that support ovulation). Because of this, IUI has a one-in-ten chance of resulting in multiples, due to the increased likelihood of more than one egg being released during a month's menstrual cycle. Clomid can also cause such, ahem, *pleasant* side effects such as nausea and vomiting, abdominal tenderness, sore breasts, headache, and abnormal vaginal bleeding. To clarify, my partner was not on any medication and, as a result, experienced no side effects. And I firmly can attest to all the side effects listed above.

Though popular culture might lead you to believe that IUI is equivalent to a turkey baster, there is more specificity involved. During IUI, a thin catheter is inserted into the vaginal opening and then through the cervical opening. Through this catheter, my partner's sperm was placed in my uterus, increasing the chances of it reaching the egg(s) in the fallopian tubes.

On the day of the procedure, my partner, Roy, was given the slightly embarrassing task of "collecting" his semen in a small, private room stocked with reading and viewing material an hour before I was led into a cold procedure room. As I lay on my back, feet in stirrups, a resident physician assured me he would have no difficulty finding my cervix as he had performed this procedure hundreds of times. After forty-five minutes of being "so close" to grasping the lip of my cervix, complete with commentary about how "they weren't kidding" in regard to the difficulty of both the location and the position of my cervix, a second doctor was asked to come in to help. Eventually my cervical lip was grasped, catheter inserted, and sperm injected. Afterward, I was told to hope for a missed period in a couple of weeks and I left the procedure room with fingers crossed, a long two weeks ahead of me.

My path to that pregnancy was not without obstacles, but it was still a relatively easy process, all things considered.

On average, a woman under the age of thirty-five will have a 10 to 20 percent chance of conceiving during the first cycle of IUI. (The good news is that with each cycle of IUI, the chances of conceiving get better!) But with the first cycle, that percentage goes down to 2 to 5 percent for women over thirty-five. It is often recommended that women under forty complete three IUI cycles before moving on to try IVF. For women over the age of forty, only one cycle is recommended.

I was fortunate to conceive on the first round of treatment. I had a positive pregnancy test on July 5 and gave birth to my daughter on April 5 the following year.

My path to that pregnancy was not without obstacles, but it was still a relatively easy process, all things considered. I had some fertility issues that were easily overcome with the first line of fertility interventions. I had a child at home and knew the joy and challenge of being a mother, something that some women, couples, and birth parents, who are in the grasp of infertility, are desperate to experience.

REFLECT
light visualization

Visualizing can be a meditative practice. Set aside ten to fifteen minutes to practice this healing light visualization. Begin by lying down in any comfortable position that allows you to relax fully. Close your eyes and begin doing a body scan to notice places you are holding any tension. Move your attention slowly through your body, feet to head, releasing any gripping or holding along the way. Then, visualize a healing, bright, warm light emanating from above. This light might be white or bright yellow or pale purple or any other color that feels distinctively healing. Imagine this light slowly washing over you, touching the tips of your toes and spreading upward through your body. Imagine this light reaching the crown of your head and radiating from there. Become aware of this light settling into the bowl of your pelvis. You can imagine the light swirling around or dropping in gently, like a cat nestling into a comfy blanket. You might also imagine feeling a sensation of warmth settle over you as the light makes contact with your body. Breathe deeply, feeling this healing light move through your body as you inhale, and then allow it to slowly dissipate as you exhale. When the light has moved through you and dissipated, come out of this visualization.

RELATE
anna's fertility story

Yoga practitioner and mom to two young boys, Anna, shares about her winding path to motherhood.

It's hard to describe the conflicting and crazy-making advice I got, unsolicited and solicited, about doing yoga while dealing with infertility from people who know nothing about yoga to reproductive endocrinologists to master yoga teachers.

"Have you tried doing yoga? It will help you relax."

"Don't do yoga, it will overstress your body! Take a three-month break."

"Meditate every day."

"You can keep up with whatever you normally do."

"Just do restorative poses."

"The restrictions are the same as pregnancy: no jumping, twisting, or core work."

"Do deep, belly-heating core work."

So many of these suggestions made me bristle. I was told to modify my practice the same way a pregnant woman should. No thanks! Another suggestion was to drop my asana practice for three months. And at the same time I was being told to blame the way I did yoga, I was also being told to meditate (which I already did nearly daily) and do restorative yoga (which I also did).

I'm not a religious person, but I imagine this is what it would feel like for an anguished believer to be told she had brought her infertility on herself by not worshiping the right way. That if she would just pray on it the right way—all the while feeling she had been forsaken by her god—she would be healed. It hurt not only to think about giving up the kind of practice I wanted. It also cut deeply because it threatened the idea that I was in touch with what my body needed through practice. And yet, despite my anger at having to throw this one last sacred refuge on the pyre, I did it. I mostly gave up asana for months to not drain my body's apparently insufficient biological resources away from the chance to reproduce.

I went deeply into Ayurveda, yoga's sister science of holistic medicine and lifestyle.

Instead of yoga asana, I went deeply into Ayurveda, yoga's sister science of holistic medicine and lifestyle. According to Ayurveda, the body has eight layers of tissue (*dhatus*): plasma, blood, muscle, fat, bone, bone marrow, nerve, and reproductive tissues. Ayurveda posits that the tissues are accessible in this order, and they break down in this order, so reproductive disorders are the result of deep imbalances. Happily for me, my path to rebalance involved eating tons of avocados, ghee, and other sumptuous fats. Once I was more balanced and I had gained a few much-needed pounds, I did an initial cleanse before my fourth IVF cycle. While the results were better (more eggs!), the embryos still weren't strong, and the cycle failed.

We started thinking about donor eggs. I thrashed emotionally harder than I ever have in my life: hating the idea, feeling it like an inevitable pull, resenting prospective egg donors, and wanting to do everything in my power to just make infertility stop. In meditation one morning, I saw myself standing in front of a waterfall. Like many of them, it had a tiny cave behind the water, a special mossy hideout. My emotions had been, as usual, racing about donor eggs. Suddenly, I was pulled into the little cave, and I sat there, cool water a shield between me and everything outside; that's when I felt it: I understood that my despair, clinging, frustration, anger, regret, and resentment were what my desire to have a child felt like. There was no joy, no positive vision in it. It was then I realized, I don't want to have kids. *I want us to be parents.* A desire to replicate my genes didn't have to drive the train; I could get what I most wanted out of parenthood without biological kids.

Our fifth IVF cycle was going to be our last one using my eggs. But I didn't get pregnant. Instead, I got told I probably had an unidentifiable condition that meant I could never have children.

The clarity of the waterfall was gone. The finality of it, the pronouncement that no matter what I did our efforts would be futile, was one of the most anguishing moments of my life. I felt so many things. One of them, particular to yoga, was the sense of confronting *abhinivesha*, "clinging to bodily life," which the *Yoga Sutras* identify as one of the obstacles to spiritual growth (*kleshas*). In all our years of trying, all the failures had pushed me from an ambivalent maybe-mom to fervent clinging to the idea that I could do this. Being told that I could never reproduce, no matter what, felt not only like a slap in the face of my agency and ability, it felt like being erased from the human family. It felt like dying in an evolutionary sense.

Along with the devastation, I felt deep relief knowing that I would never subject my body to a hormone-stimulating cycle again. I went to a workshop at Kripalu in the Berkshires of Massachusetts, and in it we were asked to talk to our bodies and tell them what they needed to hear. Immediately, without thinking, I said to my body, "I'm sorry. I'm so, so, so sorry." Not that my body couldn't get pregnant but for all the flogging she went through. I recommitted to having a sweet, kind relationship with her and nourishing her in any way she needed.

I marshaled all my resources of intention and mindfulness to create a ceremony I shared with a few family members and a friend. Together we meditated. We talked about the love for our children we hadn't been able to express publicly. We lit a candle for each of the 116 eggs that had not become our children. We grieved my genetic contribution to our future children and lit the way to welcome the idea of donor eggs.

Even as we moved on, I regained a bedrock belief in my body. I kept up my Ayurvedic diet, herbs, and self-care; I did a spring cleanse. I started doing unrestricted asana again, feeling a challenging practice as a gift and slow, contemplative practices as a comforting friend. I kept seeing a really gifted acupuncturist.

Six months later—when, after a series of setbacks, we were exploring a third prospective egg donor—I got pregnant. Just after I got pregnant, I wrote in my journal: "If this sticks and if I have this baby, I could rewrite my story as one of inevitability but that's not how it felt at the time, so I won't rewrite it into a neat and perfect story line."

Along with extraordinary good luck, I credit my acupuncturist, the physical and emotional boost from Ayurveda, my therapist, my husband for his endless support, and a few friends who supported me with the donor egg plan. And I also credit *me*: for years of work, dedication, self-care, and emotional healing. It was partially the yoga—as a holistic framework for my life. It wasn't doing or giving up specific poses or seated meditation or pranayama or Ayurveda that got me pregnant. I learned I couldn't barter these practices in exchange for a pregnancy, no matter how subtly or sophisticatedly I tried to mask the trade.

MOVE
yoga for life's stress

Yoga chitta vritti nirodha, the reminder that yoga is one path for calming our busy, buzzy minds, is at the heart of this practice. As yoga teachers, we know that we aren't just offering a workout class when we share a yoga sequence: We're designing something that marries breath and movement to offer peace, presence, and spaciousness—all with the intention of being a respite from our deep stressors. In this practice, you'll move not to "escape" the anxiety, busyness, or stress you feel, but to be present with it. You may notice a shift in your awareness of this anxiety—it may dissipate or lessen as you move your body and tune into your breathing. It may not, and that's okay too. One thing you *don't* want to do here is add to your sense of stress if you don't get the desired "results" from your yoga practice. Remind yourself that however your emotions feel before, during, and after this practice, your body is getting to move and open and stretch. That is so valuable on its own.

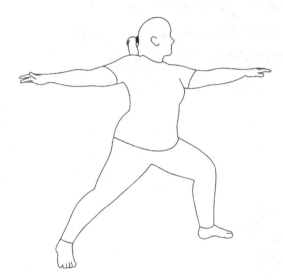

Warrior 2

Start at the top of your mat, and step your right foot back, taking a wide stance. With your left foot perpendicular to the front edge of your mat, your right foot angled slightly inward, begin to bend your left knee. Bring your arms up to shoulder height and extend outward from the center of your chest. Turn your gaze toward your left fingertips. Even in this fierce pose, is there a place where you can soften? Notice if any of the muscles in your face are working when they needn't be, and invite your jaw, cheeks, and forehead to relax.

Exalted warrior

Keeping the sides of your waist long and your legs and feet in the same position, lower your right hand down the length of your right leg as you lift your left hand upward. Rest your right hand lightly on your back leg, keeping your front body open and spacious. Allow your gaze to drift upward and continue to sink into your left leg while remaining strong in your right leg.

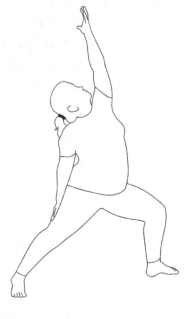

Side angle pose

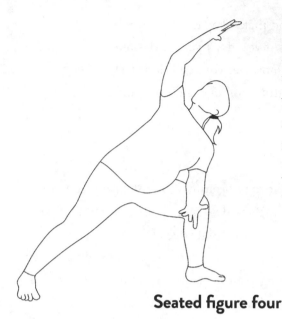

Maintaining the position of your legs, bring your torso upright and lower your left forearm to your thigh, or your fingertips to a block or to the floor. Extend your right arm alongside your ear such that the line from your right foot to your right fingertips forms a diagonal line.

Repeat the three previous poses with your right foot forward and your left foot at the back of your mat.

Seated figure four

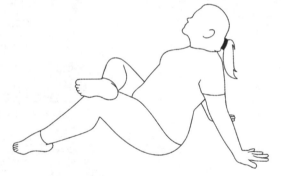

From side angle pose on the right side, step back into downward-facing dog. Turn your gaze toward the front of your mat and walk your feet forward. Have a seat, and bend your knees, placing your feet on the floor. Cross your left ankle over the top of your right knee. Resist your left knee away from your chest. You may rock your legs a little side to side if that feels good. Repeat this pose with your right ankle crossed over your left knee.

Happy baby

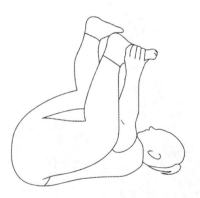

Come onto your back. Hug both knees into your chest. Separate your knees to either side and draw them out wide and toward your chest. Lift your feet upward, holding either your ankles or your feet. It should look as if you are doing an upside-down squat. You might choose to be still or to rock side to side.

As with all yoga practices, we encourage you to rest in savasana after this practice.

REFLECT
affirmations to confer strength in the face of anxiety

Affirmations can be little phrases you use in your mind in moments of insecurity and fear. You can also chant them as mantras or repeat them out loud. Here are some phrases you can practice in your car on your way to doctors' appointments, in waiting rooms, right before bed, or in any moments of high anxiety.

I am whole as I am.
Nothing has to happen now.
I am open to listen.
I am open to life.
Om mani padme hum.

Chanting or repeating this last one, *om mani padme hum,* a Tibetan Buddhist mantra which translates to reverence for the jewel in the lotus, can be a reminder that you already possess all that you need: innate wholeness and wisdom.

WISDOM
a perinatal mental health specialist's thoughts on infertility

Samantha Hellberg, PhD candidate in Clinical Psychology, specializing in perinatal mood, offers her thoughts on how challenging this time can be.

Infertility can have a profound impact on our mental health and well-being. Fertility-related challenges represent a multifaceted stressor. It is not uncommon for individuals to experience emotional, sexual, spiritual, and identity challenges during infertility. Indeed, the majority of individuals report experiencing significant stress related to infertility, and research has shown as many as one in two women facing infertility may experience depression or anxiety. The lack of awareness around the impacts of infertility on psychological well-being can lead to stigma, isolation, and difficulties accessing mental health support. If you are experiencing infertility-related stress or noticing changes in your mood or behavior amidst infertility, you are not alone. Here are a few ideas to get you started as you develop your own infertility care plan.

Often, when we are experiencing stress, we have the urge to shut down, withdraw from others, or stop doing the things we love. Consider instead turning toward—rather than away from—what's important to you. It can be helpful to stay connected with loved ones and friends and continue to do things that give you joy and help you feel effective.

In challenging times, we can also turn to coping strategies that might help us feel better in the short-term but make things more challenging in the long-term. We might turn to food or substances to cope or try to avoid or deny the stressor. To shift this pattern, you might start by noticing how you cope with stress, and how well these strategies are working. Take note of the small things that alleviate stress and lift you up: yoga, movement, time in nature, prayer, meditation, a favorite candle, time to craft. Then see if you can build a bit more time for these things into your day. Consistency is key, and small, sustainable changes can go a long way.

Consistency is key, and small, sustainable changes can go a long way.

If you feel stuck leaning on unhelpful coping strategies or want more skills for managing stress, therapy can be helpful. Mental health professionals with training in infertility and stress can help you develop a care plan that aligns with your goals and needs. Different mental health supports are available, such as individual, group, or couples therapy, as well as medications and support groups. To start, I recommend checking that your provider has solid training in approaches backed by research. For example, acceptance- and mindfulness-based as well as cognitive-behavioral treatments have been shown to improve mental health and reduce infertility-related stress, with potential benefits for pregnancy outcomes as well.

In short, if you're struggling, know that there are things that can help. No single approach works for everyone. Rather, it's important that you do what works for you and are connected with the support you need as you navigate these challenging times. You deserve to be well.

MOVE
a sequence for courage

Moving blindly, not knowing what comes next or how to shape the future you want, is a precarious place to be. In this sequence, you're invited to balance, move, and dance from a place of courageous wholeheartedness. Move, twist, explore, and be fully in your body, moving with fierceness, and bravery. Alexandra loves this playful and fierce sequence; it reminds her of her innate strength and power! Two blocks are useful for this practice.

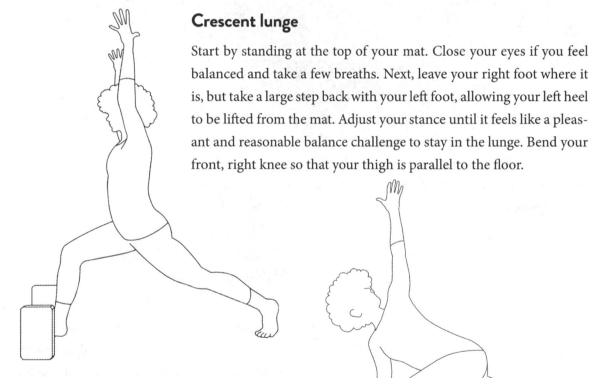

Crescent lunge

Start by standing at the top of your mat. Close your eyes if you feel balanced and take a few breaths. Next, leave your right foot where it is, but take a large step back with your left foot, allowing your left heel to be lifted from the mat. Adjust your stance until it feels like a pleasant and reasonable balance challenge to stay in the lunge. Bend your front, right knee so that your thigh is parallel to the floor.

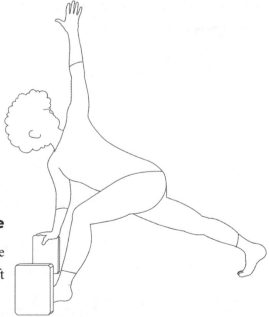

Revolved crescent lunge

From crescent lunge, lower your right hand to the floor or a block, pivoting your chest toward your left knee. Continue to extend your left arm upward.

Warrior 2

Rise slowly from revolved crescent lunge, and as you do, pivot your torso to the left, drop your back left heel down, and draw your arms parallel to the floor: arrive in Warrior 2.

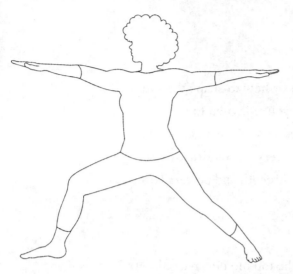

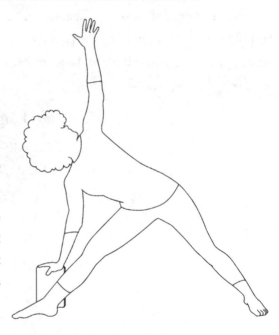

Triangle

Lower your right hand down to the floor or a block, and allow your right leg to straighten. Continue to find a soft bend in your right knee so your knee is not locked straight. Extend your left arm upward, and trust the space behind you, bringing your rib cage and hips toward alignment with each other.

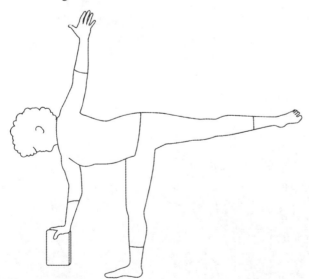

Half-moon pose

From triangle pose, gently bend your front knee to spring your back foot off the ground, coming to balance. Use your right hand as support on the ground, placing it diagonally and to the right of the front of your mat. Extend your left arm upward again, and engage the muscles of your back leg, flexing your foot. Your gaze can stay down, turned to the side, or you can even lift your gaze upward to follow your left arm.

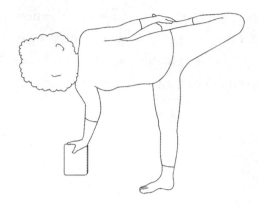

Half-moon with a bind

From your balancing half-moon pose, slowly bend your left knee, bringing your left foot toward your left hand. If you don't make that connection, that's just fine: It's pretty courageous to stretch and reach! If you do make the connection, press your foot or ankle into your hand, creating tension and stretch.

Repeat this sequence on the second side, with your left leg as the forward leg.

BREATHE
balancing breath

Alternate-nostril breathing, or *nadi shodhana*, is another breath that has been shown to decrease anxiety and increase feelings of calm and equanimity. And isn't that much-needed now as you weather the unknown during this part of the journey? To practice this breathing technique, sit somewhere you feel comfortable and supported and, using your right hand, place your thumb gently on your right nostril and your middle and ring fingers gently on your left nostril. Rest your index finger on the bridge of your nose or in the center of your forehead. For a few breaths, notice how it feels to have those fingers lightly resting on your nose, without closing off the air flow on either side. When you're ready, close off your left nostril as you breathe in through your right nostril. Invite your breath to be full and, at the top of your inhalation, take a brief pause with both nostrils gently closed. Open your left nostril and slowly exhale out this side. As you take in your next breath, keep your left nostril open and breathe in through the left side. Once again, close both nostrils and pause. Open the right side of your nose and slowly exhale. Repeat this breath sequence for as long as it feels good, working up to several minutes.

As with any breath practice (or mantra or yoga pose!) offered in this book, if it doesn't feel good to you, don't do it. Although *nadi shodhana* has the benefit of helping many people feel more grounded and balanced, closing a nostril can bring up feelings of claustrophobia. If you are experiencing any sort of nasal congestion, alternate-nostril breathing can be challenging. Instead, try deeper, slower breathing in and out through your nose or mouth for a few minutes. Anytime you tune into your breath and slow it down, allowing it to be the center of your attention, you are initiating calmness for your mind and body.

MOVE
sequence for restfulness and renewal

In times that feel outside your control (like right now, on this uncertain path to parenthood), it's helpful to feel like you're *doing* something. In a lot of wisdom traditions, including Ayurveda, those of us who are planners and doers are prescribed the opposite in order to find balance. So if you're a doer, find equanimity by making sure you also create ample space to rest. If *savasana* is the hardest part of yoga, we're talking to you here. This sequence asks you to do a lot of nothing. And that doing nothing is really doing something: It's giving your mind and body a chance to know they don't have to be on, planning, preparing, figuring out your next move, step, or appointment. Before you begin, lower your lighting and gather a cozy blanket, an eye pillow or washcloth, and a couch cushion or yoga bolster.

Legs up the wall

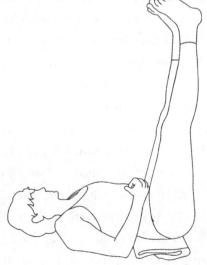

Move your mat so that the short front edge is parallel with the wall. Rest your seat as close as possible to the wall, sitting parallel to it, and then pivot and draw your legs up the wall as you lie down on your back. You can rest flat on your mat, or you can tuck a blanket under your hips and pelvis. You can also pull a blanket on top of you to feel extra cozy. You might decide to cover your eyes here with your eye pillow or washcloth. If extending your legs straight feels like effort, bend your knees, plant your feet on the wall, and drop your knees out to the sides. Rest here for many, many breaths.

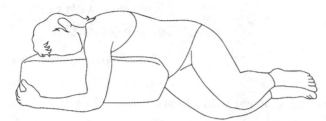

Side-lying bolster rest

Place your bolster centered on your mat, parallel. Sit perpendicular to the bolster, with your right hip pressed against the end of it, and your knees dropped to the same direction. Turn your chest to face the bolster, and then lay your belly and chest onto the bolster. Your arms can "hug" it on either side. You can turn your head in either direction—choose what feels most comfortable. If you'd like, you can tuck a blanket between your knees and thighs. Stay here for as long as you'd like and then switch sides to do the pose again, this time with your left hip against it.

Supine bound angle pose

Lie on your back in the center of your mat. Tuck your blanket under your seat and hips. Bend your knees, draw your feet together, and open your knees to either side, creating a diamond shape with your legs. Adjust your blanket to support your outer hips. Linger here.

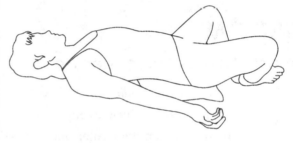

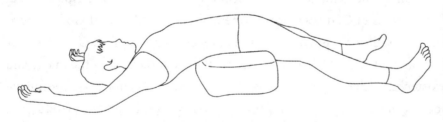

Supported bridge pose

Place your bolster centered on your mat, perpendicular. Sit on your bolster, and then lower your torso down, so that your upper back, shoulders and head are on the floor and only your pelvis remains elevated on the bolster. You can bend your knees, and plant your feet down, or you can stretch your legs out long. Your arms might go out into a T shape or you could place your arms into a V shape, more parallel to your head.

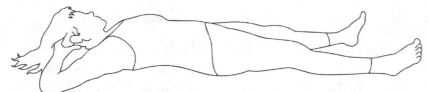

**Savasana with partner
or self-assists**

Choose your favorite savasana shape: maybe lying flat
on your back, maybe with a bolster under your knees, maybe with a blanket over your body, maybe
with an eye pillow or washcloth over your eyes. Be picky about your comfort. Snuggle up and take
time to make adjustments until you're cozy and secure. If you have a partner, ask them to sit near your
head and gently rub your head and neck for at least a full minute. If you're taking this savasana solo,
take a minute or so to rub the back of your neck, the ridge at the base of your skull, and then your
whole head, massaging your scalp with your fingers. Eventually, once you feel settled, rest here for at
least seven minutes.

WISDOM
the practice of surrendering

Ishvara pranidhana translates to surrendering to the divine. It is the last of the yoga
niyamas—the principles of personal observance. Ishvara pranidhana is a reminder that
there is something greater than yourself. If you have a faith or religious tradition that
you follow, then this may be an easy philosophy to put into practice. This idea is echoed
in other philosophies and faith traditions, including Christianity. The Apostle Paul
wrote, "The foolishness of God is wiser than men; and the weakness of God is stronger than men." This sentiment provides a sense of relief for many of us. Our desire for
control simply cannot be: It is thwarted by our smallness in the face of the magic and
mystery of existence. In the poem "Tripping Over Joy" by the Islamic mystic Rumi, he
tells us that our existence is a great chess game; the wise saint is laughing at God's great
moves in the game, saying, "I surrender," while those who are less wise still believe they
have "a thousand serious moves."

As you make your way through the ups and downs of fertility, we know that surrendering may be the last thing you want to do: Perhaps it feels like you have already
surrendered so much. Surrendering isn't a force field against pain. Surrendering is a
signifier that you trust the process. When you surrender, you turn your own will over
to a deeper, truer wisdom—however you define that for yourself.

yoga for life's stress

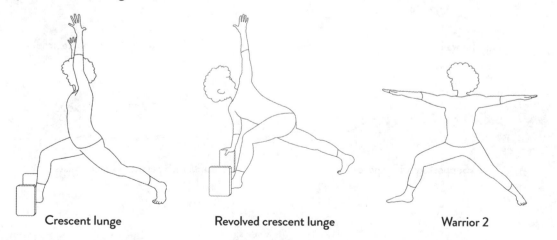

Warrior 2

Exalted warrior

Side angle pose

Seated figure four

Happy baby

a sequence for courage

Crescent lunge

Revolved crescent lunge

Warrior 2

a sequence for courage (continued)

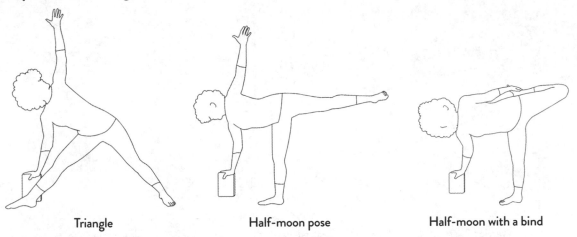

Triangle

Half-moon pose

Half-moon with a bind

sequence for restfulness and renewal

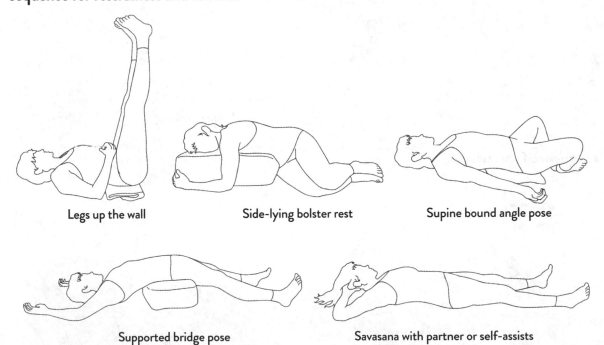

Legs up the wall

Side-lying bolster rest

Supine bound angle pose

Supported bridge pose

Savasana with partner or self-assists

Part Two

pregnancy

Chapter Three

trimester one: you're pregnant? you're pregnant!

First of all, we are so, so excited for you. We both remember the blissfully shocking moment of the positive pregnancy test, sharing with trusted family and friends, the sweet secret carried around for a while before the more public announcement that our lives were about to change in permanent and impossible-to-imagine ways. After all, being pregnant means you're steering your life into a new, unknown world, and no matter how much you read, how much information you gather, how many moms and birth parents you talk to, there are parts of pregnancy, birth, and motherhood that will remain a mystery until they are lived experiences for you.

If you identify as a woman, this may feel like a sacred moment of femininity; the culmination of many years spent with tampons, cups, pads, as your body cycled through gearing up for this very scenario again and again. Pregnancy is such a paradox: Many of us spend years trying to prevent it, some of us spend years trying to capture it, and even when it comes, there may be an entire swath of emotions: many celebratory, and some emotions of sadness, grief, or fear. If this isn't your first pregnancy, then you may have lots of feelings or reflections on your previous experience(s). If your pregnancy happened quickly, or was a surprise, it may feel like a blur of emotions are hitting you:

joy and fear, intermingled. There is no right way to feel now, and how you feel is not only influenced by your past experiences, but by your upbringing, your own intergenerational love and trauma, and, of course, the cocktail of hormones already flowing through you, which certainly influences more than science really understands.

It's helpful to remember that the human condition is one that is both unique and familiar: Your experiences and emotions are probably echoed by millions of mothers and birth parents. But sometimes it's challenging to see that, especially if you are one of the first (or last) in your community of friends or family to have children. One way that prenatal yoga can help is by offering community: Of course, in this particular iteration of yoga, we mean quite literally that you should attend a group prenatal yoga class. You can usually find a class at your local studio if you live in a yoga-robust area. If not, don't discount the value of online connection. Prenatal classes abound online (we offer them!), and you'll probably be amazed by how much you look forward to seeing and connecting with others who are also in this phase of life. Unlike typical group yoga classes, most prenatal classes begin with a check-in, so you get to know a little about the students in your class. We've loved seeing class communities grow and prenatal students connect with one another outside the class setting. It's a great way to feel as though you are part of a powerful coterie of others during a time that can sometimes otherwise seem a little isolating.

Yoga has been shown to reduce stress and help with anxiety and depression.

Yoga has been shown to reduce stress and help with anxiety and depression. It can improve sleep and increase the strength, flexibility, and endurance of muscles needed for childbirth (not to mention those needed during the forty-plus weeks of actual pregnancy!). A compilation of multiple studies of pregnant people who practice yoga show improved outcomes in many important areas related to labor and delivery. In fact, some recent studies have shown that expectant parents who routinely practiced prenatal yoga on a weekly basis were more likely to have a vaginal birth. In addition, labor was, on average, two hours shorter for folks who had practiced yoga during pregnancy.

Aside from the benefit of community and the data we have on labor and delivery outcomes, yoga offers you a chance to have time with yourself. If this is your first pregnancy, the practice of yoga gives you ample room to start the practice of listening to your intuition and making space for your deeper self. If you already have children at home, yoga can provide the time and space (and quiet!) to connect both with yourself and with your new baby. Whether you're in a yoga class with a teacher guiding you or you are moving alone on your mat, there are pockets of silence, opportunities for stillness, and chances for moving meditation. You get to show up and be with yourself, listening to your own needs; this practice will serve you through labor and into motherhood.

One other intersection between yoga and pregnancy is that in both experiences, you get to know your body better and you get to watch your body shift, change, and respond to exerted forces. Yoga gives you ample opportunity to get acclimated with your changing body outside of the typical movement you might do in daily life. It's one thing to experience the sensation of your growing belly as you put on your regular work pants; it's another to notice it when you explore twisting in a seated position in a yoga routine.

There's a relationship between your yoga practice and your awareness of your body. Krysten Spurrier, pelvic floor occupational therapist says, "In the clients that do yoga I see a lot more body awareness and calming energy. I think the inner core stability and breathing education that you can receive from yoga is very beneficial to your pelvic floor." Yoga offers a way for you to know yourself, spiritually, but also viscerally and tangibly.

WISDOM
pregnancy in the first trimester: so, like, what's happening in your body?

The first trimester of your pregnancy is weeks one through twelve. Fertilization occurs around the second week. Some women and birth parents can tell that they're pregnant fairly immediately—we've heard anecdotes that some birthing people can literally feel the implantation of the fertilized egg on their uterine wall! For others, a missed period is the first indication. Some of the first signs of pregnancy may include sore breasts, fatigue (oh, so much fatigue), nausea, aversion to smells, and, for some of us, aversion to certain foods. (For both of us the idea of a leafy, green vegetable during the first few months of pregnancy was beyond repulsive. The cracker-and-pasta diet is a legitimate way to eat for a couple of months.)

In the first trimester, your body's hormones are in overdrive. Your uterus starts to expand and grow, and your body begins to produce more blood (eventually, over the course of your pregnancy, doubling your blood volume!). As the first trimester continues, your breasts might feel heavy or even tingle. If your skin is pale, you might notice more pronounced blue veins beneath the skin on your breasts.

This next first trimester possibility can feel a little scary. Uterine cramping can occur, and even a little spotting or bleeding might happen. This is most common when your fertilized egg implants into the uterine lining. But we fully get that seeing blood or feeling cramping sensations in your uterus can feel discombobulating, so it's a wise choice to check in with your doctor or midwife.

Other common experiences of the first trimester include excess saliva (likely caused by pregnancy hormones stimulating your salivary glands), a more frequent urge to pee (more fluid in your body and also the uterus growing and pressing against its neighbor in your pelvis, your bladder), and libido changes—the idea of sex might be about as enticing as a kale salad. Another unfortunate first trimester complaint is constipation and other digestive issues.

Pregnancy, like parenting, is both extremely universal and entirely personal.

Of course, you may not have any of the symptoms we mentioned so far! Some folks are lucky enough to go through the first trimester with no nausea at all while others of us may keep a little trash can next to our beds, like an altar to the gods of antiemetics. Pregnancy can feel different for everyone. We often joke, though, that if you do an internet search for pretty much any physical ailment, oddity, or sensation and the word *pregnancy,* you'll always find *someone* to corroborate your anecdotal experience, even when medical research doesn't have an answer. Pregnancy, like parenting, is both extremely universal and entirely personal.

prenatal yoga versus regular yoga while pregnant

There is a distinct difference between classes specifically designed to serve the prenatal community and general population yoga classes you might still choose to attend during your pregnancy. Prenatal yoga teachers have an extensive understanding of pregnancy and the needs of pregnant bodies. Because yoga is often an exercise practice designated as safe by the medical community, prenatal yoga tends to attract a broad swath of students to the practice. The practice prenatal yoga teachers offer must fit the varying needs of all prenatal students. These classes tend to skew gentler, with some additive strengthening poses and movements, applicable breath work, and a community component.

Taking a non-natal yoga class while pregnant is a different experience, and it is entirely up to you whether you disclose your pregnancy. Some yoga teachers have a depth of knowledge that covers the perinatal period, and many have given birth themselves. That said, yoga training programs are not required to cover prenatal teaching, and some don't. This will likely impact the teacher more than it will you, armed with the information that you know what's best for you, what feels right, and what doesn't.

RELATE

Prenatal yoga students offer thoughts on why group prenatal classes have been useful to them during their own pregnancies.

Carly, mom to two toddlers and eight months pregnant

Prenatal yoga has been an extremely important part of all three of my pregnancies. Physically it has helped tremendously with the various aches and pains that come with pregnancy, and emotionally, the experience has been invaluable. Attending prenatal yoga class not only does wonders for my sore body, but the social/emotional element really revives my soul on a weekly basis. It is incredibly encouraging to be among other women who are experiencing the ups and downs of this motherhood journey, and I truly don't know if I could survive this final and most difficult pregnancy without the class.

Natalia, mom to a four-week-old

I wanted to practice yoga in a way that was safe during pregnancy and mindful of my growing belly. The practice was supportive and super rejuvenating, but the most important piece was the connection and community built with other women going through the same experience. Being able to hear and learn from others about their challenges and fears or celebrate their successes, while also sharing my own, was incredibly validating and supportive. Prenatal yoga classes were the highlight of my week during pregnancy.

Brittany, thirty-one weeks pregnant

Prenatal yoga has been extremely helpful for my pregnancy. My first two pregnancies ended in early miscarriage, so the third time around I was hesitant to embrace my pregnancy until I got past the worrisome first trimester. I started prenatal yoga at thirteen weeks. I am now thirty-one weeks along, and prenatal yoga has helped me through this process both physically and mentally. I've discovered that yoga doesn't have to be something that pushes me to the limit and makes me sweat buckets, but yoga can also be about slowing down and meeting your body where it is in the moment. I've also discovered that yoga is more than an insular experience and that it can foster a powerful sense of community. I don't come to class just for the stretching and mental cleansing, I now also come for the people.

WISDOM
practicing yoga while pregnant:
truths and misconceptions about what's safe

Lyz Lenz, author of *Belabored: A Vindication of the Rights of Pregnant Women*, says, "A uniting experience of American pregnancy is receiving the list of things you're forbidden from putting in your body." Practically from the very moment of conception, books, apps, elders, colleagues, friends, websites, and every other possible source around you is conspiring to make sure you're aware of all the things that can go wrong, all the ways you can mess up, all the things that are unsafe, and all the things that you have already done wrong that imperil your baby. Is it any wonder that there's fear connected to pregnancy, birth, and laboring? Fearmongering often sells things (books, unneeded pregnancy and baby gear), and having a fearful group of women and birthing people certainly lends itself to patriarchal control. To feel confident and courageous in the face of all this alarmism is to shake off the fear and find freedom in your own body and trust in your own intuition.

In her book, *Poser*, Claire Dederer, in discussing her love of yoga, dismisses prenatal yoga as a class with a "bunch of pregnant women, rolling around on the ground, farting." While she's not completely wrong (finding freedom in your body means embracing its needs, be they muscular, mental, or digestive!), yoga while pregnant doesn't require your body to slow down, be stuck exclusively on the floor, or be relegated only to restorative and gentle practices. Bodies are strong, pregnant bodies not excluded. Anyone who has ever given birth will attest to the mental and physical fortitude required to bring another life into this world. In addition to allowing space for rest and restoration, a yoga practice during pregnancy can also help to develop the strength so necessary and inherent to the act of giving birth.

Of course, our suggestions for practicing yoga during pregnancy should not take the place of any specific instructions provided by your care provider. Everyone's pregnancy is different, and if your pregnancy has some special needs, please attend to those needs. Later in this chapter we will discuss some more common pregnancy complications and whether there is any need to modify your practice as a result.

Here are some frequently asked questions from our students about what is and what isn't okay for them to do during pregnancy, at least as far as yoga is concerned. We hope it dispels some of the mistruths that are often bandied about when pregnant folks are within earshot.

common FAQs about pregnancy and yoga

Can twisting cause problems with implantation or harm the baby?

During the first trimester, your developing child is well below the abdominal organs, protected in the uterus, which is safely ensconced within the bones of the pelvis. Twisting when implantation is most likely (around the third or fourth week of pregnancy, about six to twelve days after ovulation occurs) will have no impact on the success of that occurrence: you aren't twisting your uterus, after all, which is still securely in your pelvis.

Another common concern is that twisting could compress the placenta, causing a deficiency in the blood and oxygen supply to the uterus. Compression of the placenta is highly unlikely, too. The placenta isn't fully formed until well into the second trimester, when twists begin to become awkward and uncomfortable. At that point, your uterus has risen out of your pelvis and is protecting its contents well. If closed twists (twisting toward an obstruction, usually your leg) are still possible for you, brief compression of your internal organs, your baby, and your placenta won't cause any harm. When closed twists begin to feel uncomfortable, open twists (twisting away from an obstruction) are a great option.

Can I lie on my stomach or do prone poses?

Sure! But will you want to? Chances are, the idea of placing any pressure on your front body will become repulsive and uncomfortable at some point in your pregnancy. Until that point, if you want to lie on your stomach, go for it. In our prenatal classes, we don't teach any poses that place direct weight on the belly or chest because we teach a range of pregnant folks, from those who are in the early weeks (and still feel comfortable stretched out on their bellies) to birthing people who have passed their due date. We teach to every prenatal person in our classes, so we skip the belly-down poses. But because prone poses and heart-opening poses are a pathway to opening the front of your body, you may miss your body's ability to lie facedown. There are supportive modifications that will allow for a similar experience, and you will find examples of these in the MOVE sequence called Common Modifications for Your Practice in Chapter 4.

What about my back?

You may have heard that lying on your back (particularly in the third trimester) is something to avoid. As your body mass grows because the size of your baby, placenta, and blood volume increase, there is more weight that can press down on the inferior vena cava, the largest vein in your body. This vein collects blood from your belly, pelvis, and lower extremities and returns that blood to your heart to receive oxygen. For some women and birthing people, inferior vena cava compression syndrome occurs when the (now-heavy) uterus compresses this vein when they lie flat. This can cause shortness of breath, nausea, light-headedness, dizziness, or a feeling of discomfort or anxiety. Some pregnant folks never notice it at all, but some do.

While it's unlikely to cause any issues for your growing baby before it causes personal discomfort to you, it's generally recommended that pregnant people avoid lying on their back in the third trimester. Lying on your back for brief intervals is fine, and medical professionals caution that you should not worry if you wake up to discover you have accidently been sleeping on your back for a short time. But because there is some research that suggests routinely lying on your back can cause larger issues, side sleeping is a better option. In yoga classes, take savasana on your side or use a bolster as a ramp to elevate your upper body.

I practice yoga at a heated studio. Is this okay?

Heat in excess of 102° F has been shown to potentially cause neural tube (an embryo's precursor to the central nervous system, including the brain) defects when a pregnant person is exposed to these temperatures in the early weeks of pregnancy. Although there have been no specific studies done in regard to hot yoga, for the same reasons that pregnant people are encouraged to avoid saunas and hot tubs, if your heated studio reaches temperatures of 102 and higher, it's probably best to avoid attending until you've discussed it with your care provider.

Can I do pranayama practices that involve breath holding?

The common standard of practice for many years was to recommend against any breathing practices that could possibly cause the restriction of oxygen access to your baby. It's unlikely that brief breath holding in pranayama has any impact on the oxygen flow to your baby. If these breath practices are a normal part of your practice, and you feel comfortable doing them, they're perfectly safe. If you feel dizzy or out of breath while practicing them, that's a good signal your body might be more amenable to a gentler breathing practice.

I love backbends, but I am wondering if I can continue to practice them throughout pregnancy?

During pregnancy, there is a slightly increased risk of lower back injury or muscle strain because of the extra weight on the lower back and the increased instability of the joints of the pelvis. If you've never done an intense backbend before, now might not be the time to introduce them. If they feel strong and empowering in your body, continue to pay attention and enjoy the opening of your front body. Later in the chapter, as we mentioned above, we will introduce some front body-opening possibilities that tend to feel good to most pregnant bodies.

I've heard that going upside down can be dangerous during pregnancy. Is this true?

The biggest challenge doing inversions can be the inconsistency in balance present during pregnancy. Balance gets trickier during pregnancy because of our rapidly shifting body weight and, as a result, our changing center of gravity. If you have an established headstand/handstand/going upside-down practice, there is no medical reason to discontinue if it feels good. If you do decide to practice balancing inversions while pregnant, consider having a wall or a supportive and experienced spotter nearby. And if you didn't have an inversion practice prior to getting pregnant, for reasons of balance and fall risk, this is not the time to start.

Am I supposed to avoid doing core work during pregnancy?

Your core is an essential part of the strength required to labor and give birth. A strong core during pregnancy is a very good thing! Connecting to and staying aware of the transverse abdominis (TA)—the muscle that sheaths your torso like a corset—is particularly important, as the TA forms a kind of boundary for the rest of your front body. As your belly expands forward, the rectus abdominis muscles will separate at some point. Having a strong side body (your oblique muscles) can be beneficial as your side waist serves as a container for your lower torso. The *rectus abdominis* muscles (the infamous "six-pack" muscles) are the muscles people are often referring to when they advise against core work during pregnancy. By week thirty-six of pregnancy, all birthing people will experience this separation of the *linea alba* connective tissue that runs directly through the center of rectus abdominis. This gap that occurs is called *Diastasis Rectus Abdominis* or *Diastasis Recti* (DR), and we'll talk a little more about it in Chapter 10. While there isn't good research on what causes DR, it makes good sense to avoid movements that create more pressure on the front of the abdomen. Generally, that means we avoid doing sit-ups, crunches, boat pose in yoga, or any crunch-like movement. But there's plenty of good core work to be done! See the MOVE sequence Safe Core for Pregnant Bodies, later in this chapter.

Is it okay to get my heart rate up during movement activities?

Yes. Old research suggested that having a high heart rate during pregnancy could be problematic. But it's not. In your mother's pregnancy, it was likely recommended to her that her heart rate stay below 140 beats per minute. In recent years, experts have shown that there is no "unsafe" heart rate number, and, in fact, heart-rate-raising exercise is recommended for pregnant people. Still, moderation is key, so you can probably skip your high-intensity interval training class—there is no need to exercise to the point of being out of breath and unable to talk. Do prenatal yoga instead.

MOVE
sequence for fatigue

The most common complaint of the first trimester is fatigue. A gentle yoga practice can help boost your energy. We promise it helps even when (especially when) it is one of the last things you feel like doing. So often, we hear from our students that they had to drag themselves to yoga class but are so grateful that they did because they feel so much better. The movement included in this sequence is gently energizing—it opens both the front and the back chain of your body and invites spinal movement and spaciousness. Depending on the day and how you're feeling, you could practice the gentler versions, or you could practice the more challenging versions. You might want a blanket for this sequence.

Standing forward fold hang

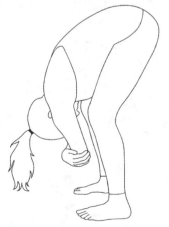

Come to your mat, and then fold forward, allowing your knees to bend as much as you'd like. Hang and dangle. You might sway side to side. You might bring your hands to either elbow. You could even take your hands behind your back, or clasp your palms behind your back and raise your hands upward. Explore what feels good here for several rounds of breath.

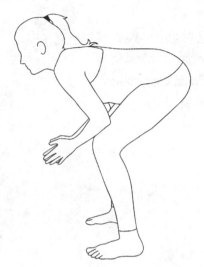

Modified standing forward fold

You can practice this pose instead of or after the previous pose. Come to your mat, and fold forward until you can prop your forearms on your upper thighs. Allow your knees to bend any degree that helps you ascertain this pose and feel comfortable. Here again, you can sway your hips, gently bend one knee and then the other, or even drop your chin toward your chest. Again, explore how you'd like to move here or settle into stillness for several rounds of breath.

Seated heart opener

Sit with your legs in front of you, knees bent, feet on the floor. Bring your hands behind your back, fingers pointed toward your seat. Roll your shoulders onto your back, and lift your heart upward. If it feels good, lift your chin too. Hold for several rounds of breath, emphasizing your exhale.

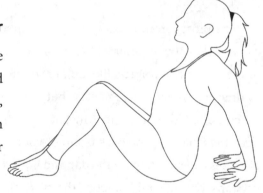

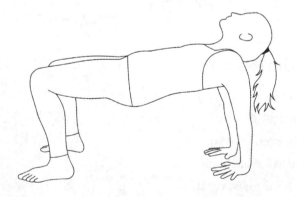

Reverse table

You can practice this pose instead of or after the previous pose. Set up similarly as in the seated heart opener, but this time press the floor away, lifting your seat, so that you are supporting your body with just your hands and feet. Notice that the muscles of your seat (your glutes) are supporting you, and intentionally engage them.

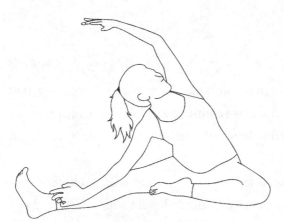

Revolved head-toward-knee pose

Sit on the floor. Extend your right leg out toward the right. Bend your left knee and tuck your left foot toward your right inner thigh. Settle your right hand on the inside of your right leg, palm facing out. Take a full breath in, and as you exhale slide your right hand down your leg toward your foot, allowing your body to side bend toward the right. When you have settled into this side bend, sweep your left arm alongside your left ear, so that your left arm and right leg are parallel. Rotate your chest upward. Stay for several breaths and then repeat this pose with your left leg out and your right foot tucked in.

Child's pose

Come on to hands and knees and take your knees as wide as you would like. Lower your chest and belly to the floor until your head touches the mat. Stretch your arms in front of you, elbows up or down. Rest here.

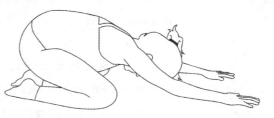

Cat pose to child's pose and back

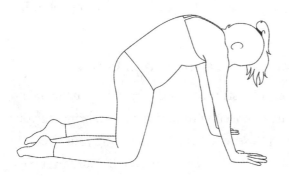

Rise from child's pose to hands and knees and round your spine, dropping your chin toward your chest. From here, play between cat pose and then back to child's pose. You can lower slowly from cat pose to child's pose, maybe swaying your hips or exploring any interesting sensations in your lower back along the way. Play between these shapes for multiple breaths, eventually resting again in child's pose to end your practice.

MOVE
sequence for nausea

First, we are so sorry. Nausea is one of the evolutionary remnants of pregnancy that we're hoping the human body will figure out as we continue along in the Anthropocene. For now, it's the second most common complaint, after fatigue, for people in their first trimester of pregnancy.

Nausea likely occurs as a result of increased levels of a hormone called *human chorionic gonadotropin* (HCG), which starts being produced shortly after a fertilized egg attaches to your uterus. For most birth parents, nausea is reduced or completely subsides in the second trimester, but for some it is a pregnancy-long journey. Sometimes this side effect is accompanied by vomiting, sometimes not; regardless, we know it is always miserable. We are hopeful that you have found some non-yogic means of support for your nausea—small, high-carb meals (all the crackers), ginger candies, peppermint tea, and eating a little before you even get out of bed in the morning might all provide some relief.

In offering this sequence, we realize that the idea of moving your body in any way may feel like enough to make you sick. Let us be the first to give you permission to not move if that is what is best for you. Still, we often found that slow and deliberate movement and breathing practices were helpful in subduing that horrible "low-grade stomach bug" feeling so familiar to those first twelve weeks. For this sequence, it's helpful to have a pillow or bolster, as well as a block (or substitute for a block), for the following poses.

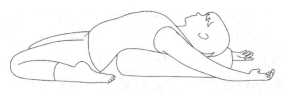

Hero's pose, arms alongside ears

Place a bolster toward the back of your mat, and come to kneeling toward the front, bringing your knees close together and separating your heels hip distance apart. Settle your seat in between your heels and lie back over the bolster. If your lower back feels tight or uncomfortable, place an extra blanket or blankets on top of your bolster to support your upper body. Once you have reclined such that your back body is supported by the bolster, try stretching your arms alongside your ears, supported by the floor. This position can give your front body additional space and is a yoga pose most often cited for its capacity to relieve nausea.

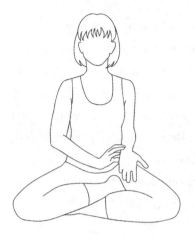

Pressure point P6

Come back up to a seated position (or stay where you are if you feel comfortable), and place your index, middle, and ring finger of your right hand at the base of your left wrist, so that the index finger is approximately in the center of the width of your forearm. Exert gentle pressure here while you take a few deep breaths in and out through your nose, pausing for a few counts at the top of your inhalation before breathing back out.

Legs on a chair

This is a variation of *viparita karani* or legs up a wall, which we explored in Chapter 2. Lie down on your back and scoot up close to a couch or chair. Lift your calves up onto the couch so that your shins are parallel to the floor. Rest here for as long as it feels good.

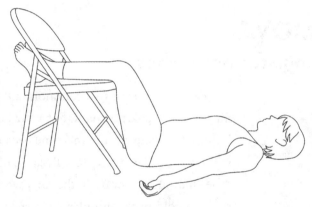

Seated, head on chair

Alternatively, or in addition to the previous pose, come to a seat and lean your forehead on a chair (a bonus if the surface of the chair is cool—metal folding chairs work great) and rest here for several rounds of breath. Lauren once rested this way for so long (she may have fallen asleep) that she ended up with a small bruise on her forehead. So, maybe not *that* long!

pregnancy

BREATHE
cool your breathing

Sitali pranayam, often referred to as "the cooling breath," is a great pranayama practice for the first trimester (or any trimester) of pregnancy and, along with deep belly breaths and nostril breathing, can assist in providing some nausea relief. To practice sitali breathing, stick your tongue out and, if you are able, make a straw-shaped roll with your tongue. If you aren't able to create that shape with your tongue, gently purse your lips instead, making a small "O" with your mouth. Breath in slowly through your tongue or your lips, as though you were sipping the air through a straw. Retract your tongue into your mouth, or soften your lips, and breathe out slowly through your nose. Repeat these five or ten times, or as many as feels good to you.

MOVE
yoga for headaches

Headaches are also a common "ailment" of the first trimester, a time in which you may not yet look pregnant, but your body certainly won't let you forget that you are. Headaches occur during this time because of changing hormones, but the rise in blood volume may play a role, too. Because of the increase of saliva and mucus, sinus headaches may also show up in the early weeks of pregnancy. When your head hurts, a dark room, a cold pack, and blessed silence might all help. Here are a few yoga tricks that may be useful, too.

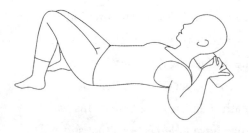

Skull and block massage

Lie down on your back with your knees bent and your feet placed solidly on the ground. Rest your inner knees together to support your lower back. Bring your block (or a tennis ball, or two tennis balls in a sock) to the back of your head, right where your spine meets your skull. Hold the block at an angle and use the long end to massage the muscles along the occipital ridge of your skull, moving your head rather than your block/ball.

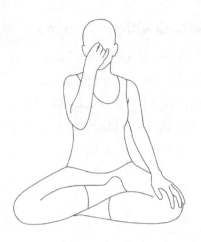

Sukhasana with nose pinch

Come up to a comfortable seated position and use your thumb, index, and middle finger to pinch the upper ridge of your nose. Take a few rounds of breath, letting go of tension in your face.

Sukhasana with rounded back

Remain seated and drop your chin to your chest. Begin to round your back, especially your upper back, and allow

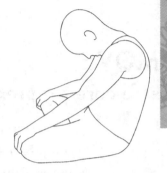

the weight of your head to be heavy. Stay here for several breaths in order for your connective tissue to have a moment to release its grip.

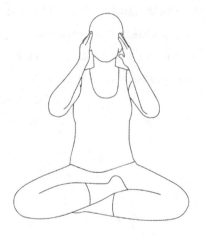

Sukhasana with temple massage

Place your index and middle fingers on your temples and massage the area in very gentle and slow circles, reversing directions after a few breaths.

Sukhasana with arm out to the side

Release your hands down to either side of your

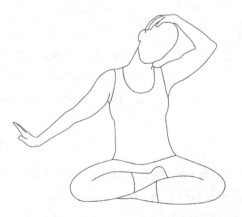

body and release your right ear toward your right shoulder. Walk your left fingertips out to the left and pause. If you'd like to intensify the stretch, lift your left hand off the floor. Play around with lifting your left arm up and notice how that

changes the quality of the stretch in the side of your neck. Explore a bit with your chin by lifting and lowering it at an angle; subtle shifts in the positioning of your head can really impact the sensation in your neck. After a few rounds of breath, bring your head back up to center and repeat on the other side, releasing your left ear toward your left shoulder and walking your right hand out to the right.

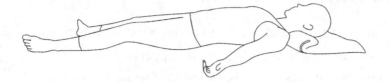

Savasana **with neck support**

Make a small roll out of a blanket or towel, large enough to support the curve of your neck. Lie down on your mat and place the rolled-up blanket behind your neck.

MOVE
safe core for pregnant bodies

Connecting to your core space during your pregnancy can be a helpful way to maintain proprioception of your changing body; even as your belly expands, contracting and engaging the muscles of your abdomen can help you understand the boundaries of your body. In yoga philosophy, the solar plexus or *manipura* chakra is around your navel, and it is the center of your personal power. Even as your body grows to encompass another little being, physical core work can help you stay connected to this powerful

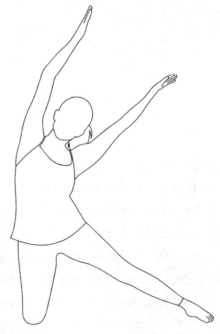

part of your body. The goal of this sequence (and core work in general during pregnancy) isn't to build your core strength, but to connect you to your preexisting core strength, so that you *remain* connected to this space in your body, even as it transforms further over the next few weeks.

Gate pose core sway

Start on hands and knees. Kickstand your right leg out to the side, and then walk your hands back to your knees until you can rise up into this one-knee down kneeling position. Make sure you feel comfortable and grounded here. With an inhale, sweep your arms overhead. With an exhale, gently sway away from your outstretched right leg toward the left. Sway far enough to

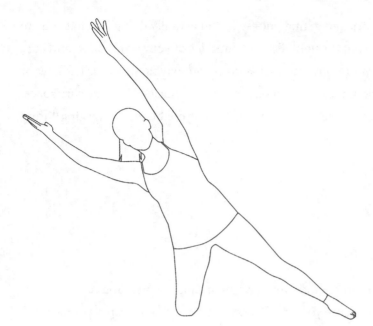

notice that you are using the muscles of your side waist and belly to support this movement into the sway and out of it. Inhale to return to center, and then exhale to sway toward your right leg, enjoying a side-body stretch. Repeat this two more times, finally swaying toward the right to stay.

Repeat this again, with your left leg out as a kickstand.

Snug baby in

Start on hands and knees. Find neutral, pointing your tailbone toward your heels and drawing your shoulders away from your ears. Take a full breath in. As you exhale, tuck your lowest ribs into your body and snug your baby farther into your belly space. Each time you breathe out, feel your core muscles tighten and engage around your expanded abdomen.

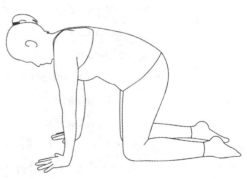

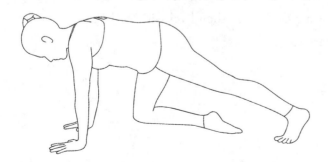

Leg out, little lift

Start on hands and knees. Extend your right leg long behind you, letting your toes stay on the ground. It may feel nice to shift your weight between your hands and outstretched leg a few times. Finally, find stillness, and snug your baby in toward your body. Draw your attention to your left knee on the mat. Tuck your left toes under. Imagine—without actually doing it—that you are about to pull your left knee up and away from the floor. Feel the muscles of your arms, back, and core engage as you gently, gently start to shift your body into that action. You may not lift your left knee at all, or you may lift it an imperceptible amount. Keep the focus on staying engaged in your core space, not on how high (or whether) you lift your knee. Explore this for multiple breaths, engaging/lifting on the exhale.

Repeat this again, with your left leg out long instead.

WISDOM
your baby is with you forever

We would be remiss not to mention miscarriage in this chapter. You don't need us to recite the statistics on it because you very likely have done that research yourself. We hope that you experience pregnancy free from any loss along the way.

Fetal-maternal microchimerism is the name for the phenomenon that occurs with every pregnancy: The tiny fetus in your body sheds cells that become part of your blood and tissues. Whether or not you carry to term, the being inside you has left an imprint on you at the cellular level. We often talk about connection or union in relation to yoga: Yoga is a union between you and your body. Yoga helps us remember that we are all made of the same life force; all of us everywhere are connected.

Microchimerism brings this idea to life. Every pregnancy you have had has been a union between your body and the life spark inside it, and every pregnancy you've had is now a part of you, in your body, in your blood, in your organs. Every woman or birthing parent who has been expectant now moves forth in their lives with the lingering energy of every possible child they have carried.

sequence for fatigue

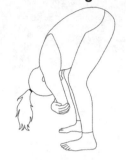

Standing forward fold hang

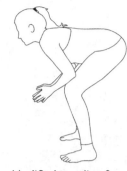

Modified standing forward fold

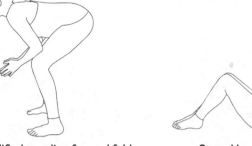

Seated heart opener

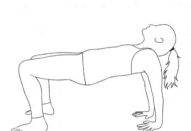

Reverse table

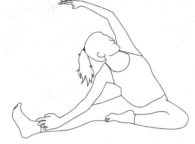

Revolved head-toward-knee pose

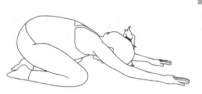

Child's pose

sequence for nausea

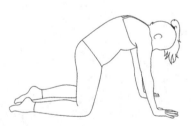

Cat pose to child's pose and back

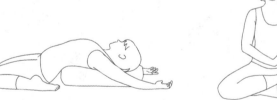

Hero's pose, arms alongside ears

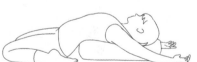

Pressure point P6

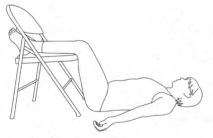

Legs on a chair

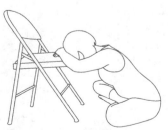

Seated, head on chair

yoga for headaches

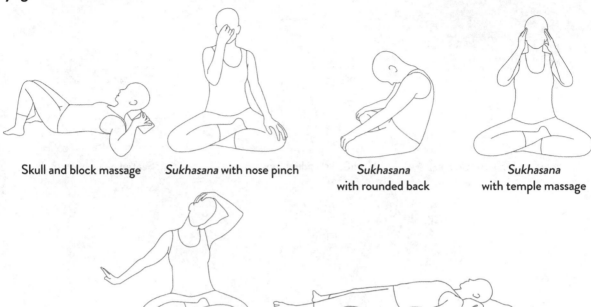

Skull and block massage

Sukhasana with nose pinch

Sukhasana
with rounded back

Sukhasana
with temple massage

Sukhasana with arm out to the side

Savasana with neck support

safe core for pregnant bodies

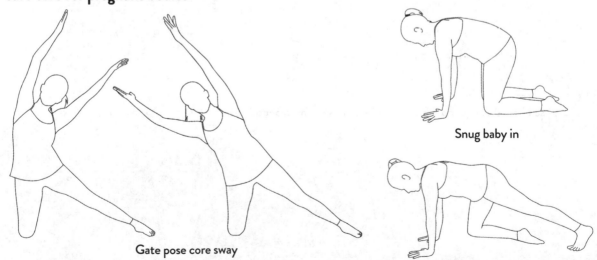

Gate pose core sway

Snug baby in

Leg out, little lift

Chapter Four

trimester two: how to breathe when a stranger asks when you're due (again)

Easily the most exciting part of the second trimester is that you're starting to look and feel pregnant (as opposed to mostly just looking like yourself, but feeling icky, depleted, and, well, weird). Unlike so many of the other huge transitions we go through in life, pregnancy announces itself to everyone: the stranger on the subway, the hostess at the restaurant, the elderly woman behind you in the checkout line. For most bodies, it's hard to hide a growing baby bump, and you might feel many different ways about that disclosure to the world.

When we started collaborating on prenatal and postpartum yoga, one thing that we both agreed on is that we did not want to market pregnancy as "precious." Undoubtedly, it is a wild, beautiful, indescribable passage of your life, and it may even be a precious experience for you. But if it's not, we want to reassure you it does not have to be. If pregnancy feels loathsome, that's okay. If pregnancy feels glorious, that's okay. If pregnancy feels sometimes loathsome and sometimes glorious, that's okay. Women are sold the idea of rose petal–filled baby showers, soft pastel blankets, and all things cuddly, but the reality is that pregnancy is a very visceral, tactile, real experience, and it can be disagreeable and harsh—and you'll still give birth to an amazing human being. Your experience of growing a child (and birthing a child) has little to do with what it will feel like to mother a child. And although the two things are related, pregnancy and parenting are two distinct seasons in life, and your feelings about them may be quite distinct, too.

This is important to keep in mind when strangers ask about your growing belly in reverent tones. If you are undeniably excited and want to share that excitement, fantastic. But your experience of pregnancy is your own, and you can politely rebuff that conversation. You may also notice that this is the trimester that somehow signifies permission to your friends and family (and those aforementioned strangers) to comment on the size, appearance, and shape of your belly. There may be speculation on how many babies you're carrying, or the sex of said babies, or whether you're carrying high or low.

Ironically, just as your pregnancy is announcing itself publicly, you may be feeling a desire to nest, move inward, and grow quieter. In yoga, the word *pratyahara* means withdrawal of senses. It's often used in the context of meditation, but it makes sense here too. In your second trimester, you may be turning inward more, moving away from the noise outside yourself. So when a stranger does ask when you're due, take a deep breath and remember this sacred, inward shifting that's occurring as you redefine your life, your relationship with yourself, your body, and your partner—and the growing life inside you. Then only answer if you want to.

WISDOM
so, what's happening in my body now?

Trimester two begins at week thirteen (when you still may not appear pregnant) and lasts until week twenty-seven (when it is fairly likely that you will have a noticeable bump). Commonly known as the "easiest" trimester of pregnancy, that may mean little to you if you're still unable to keep anything down, or if you are feeling uncomfortable in your changing body. For many, this is the time that energy begins to increase, and a good number of the challenges from the first trimester start to subside. For those of you wondering where that elusive glow of pregnancy is hiding, please know that for so many, pregnancy is a really trying and physically demanding period of life—there may be no glow at all. As one of Lauren's friends told her when she wondered why she didn't feel "amazing" in week fourteen, "You're still pregnant, after all."

That's not to say that some people don't really enjoy this trimester. Though symptoms of the first trimester don't suddenly stop the moment you cross the week thirteen threshold, they do often start to mellow out and eventually recede. Nausea (and its accompanying aversion to smells) usually eases by week sixteen. While the reason for this is not definitively known, it's likely related to the shift in hormone production. At week sixteen, pregnancy hormones are being released by the placenta and are no longer entirely systemic.

During this trimester, pregnancy and its end result often become less theoretical and more real. (Of course it always was, but our brains sometimes have a hard time fully wrapping themselves around that reality until our bellies start to protrude!) Between weeks eighteen and twenty-two you might begin to feel your baby's movement; those kicks are an incredible reminder that a baby will be arriving at the end of your pregnancy. As the weight of your body continues to change and your uterus grows, you might notice more instability in your hips and pelvis. Our friend and fellow yoga instructor, Sara, once said during prenatal yoga class that she felt fine, aside from the fact that it felt like her legs weren't attached to her body anymore.

Another impact to your lower body can be leg cramps, especially at night, along with restless legs syndrome—a condition that seems entirely unnecessary. Stretching your calves may be useful; you could also try some self-massage or gentle foam rolling. Because of the increased fluid and inflammation in the body, nasal congestion and sinus pressure are another possible symptom at this time. Have pocket tissues and a water bottle at the ready at all times.

Skin changes are common during the second trimester, too. Most birthing parents will notice a dark line running vertically down their bellies: *linea nigra*. *Chloasma* (or *melasma*) is the darker skin "pregnancy mask" that some women will get, primarily on their faces or other sun-exposed patches of skin. Hormones secreted by the placenta are thought to cause this, although there are some old wives' tales that suggest the darkening of the linea nigra and areolas are to help your baby find your breasts to nurse upon their arrival.

Round ligament pain is something we often hear about in prenatal classes. You have two of these ligaments. Along with other ligaments, the round ligaments connect your uterus to your pelvis. As your uterus gets bigger and heavier through pregnancy, the round ligaments stretch to continue to support the uterus. As a result, some pregnant people experience round ligament pain in their hips, belly, or groin. This pain may be sharp or dull, and it can be triggered when you move in a sudden way. Although this sensation can be intense, it is generally just an indication that one of the round ligaments is stretching. (After all, the ligaments start pregnancy between two and four inches long and can grow to be up to twelve inches long by the end of pregnancy!) Of course, if anything is happening in your body that is concerning you, don't hesitate to reach out to your care provider for guidance.

MOVE
common modifications for your practice

If you had a consistent yoga practice prior to becoming pregnant, you may enjoy maintaining a similar practice, or continuing to attend your regular class. Particularly in the second trimester, when some of the symptoms of the first trimester have (hopefully) resolved, but the additional weight feels manageable, it can start to feel fun to explore your familiar practices in a changing body. Many adjustments to a regular yoga practice may be fairly intuitive, but we are including some common poses below, along with adjustments for your changing body. When in doubt, *create space*. If the studio where you practice is equipped with yoga props such as blocks, blankets, and bolsters, take full advantage. If you're practicing at home or in a space without these items, use items around your home that approximate yoga props.

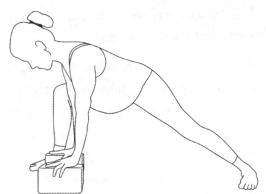

Standing poses (humble warrior)

In any standing pose, the goal is to create space and support. That means you should widen or shorten your stance as needed. In poses where your legs are apart, your back foot doesn't need to be in line with your front foot. It can be taken out to the side for a wider base of support. In lunge poses where arms are lowered toward the floor, blocks can be helpful under your hands to create more space. Additionally, your arms (and blocks) can come to the inside of your legs in order to create more space for your belly.

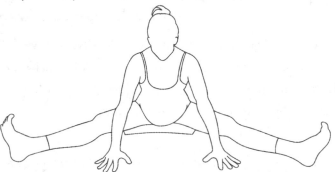

Forward folds (seated wide-legged forward fold)

In any forward fold, whether seated or standing, take your feet and legs wide enough apart to make room for your baby. In standing forward folds, blocks under your hands may be helpful for stability. In seated forward folds, a blanket under your hips can be useful in creating a little more room for your lower back and hip flexors.

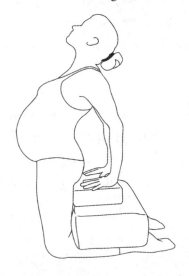

Backbends (camel with bolster and blocks on calves)

Some backbends are done prone. In these shapes, use a bolster to lift your thighs off the ground and create space for your belly. In general, you might opt to substitute gentler backbends for more intense ones. If you're in a general yoga class and the teacher offers full wheel, you might choose a gentle camel or bridge pose.

pregnancy

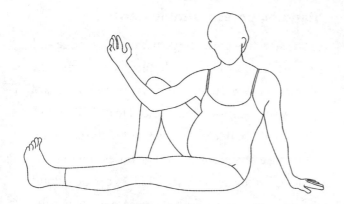

Twisting (open twist in half lord of the fishes pose)

In your first trimester, closed twists might feel fine. As your belly takes up more room, choose open twists (twisting away from an obstacle) rather than closed twists. This will allow space for your belly while still giving a sense of spinal rotation and release.

Seated hip openers (seated bound angle on cushion, block under each knee)

These types of poses are generally accessible. Not many modifications are needed for seated hip openers. Still, blocks and a blanket will often provide cushioning or allow your hips and inner thighs to open in a way that is a little gentler.

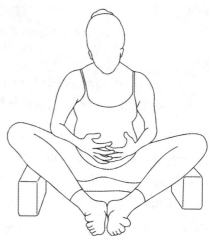

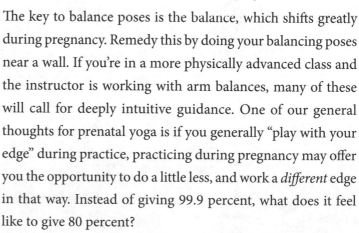

Balancing poses (tree at wall)

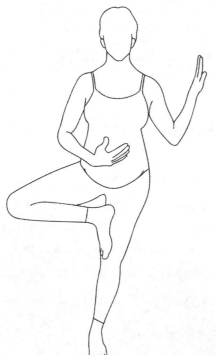

The key to balance poses is the balance, which shifts greatly during pregnancy. Remedy this by doing your balancing poses near a wall. If you're in a more physically advanced class and the instructor is working with arm balances, many of these will call for deeply intuitive guidance. One of our general thoughts for prenatal yoga is if you generally "play with your edge" during practice, practicing during pregnancy may offer you the opportunity to do a little less, and work a *different* edge in that way. Instead of giving 99.9 percent, what does it feel like to give 80 percent?

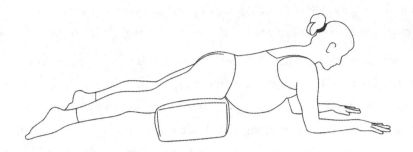

Belly-down poses (sphinx with bolster under hips)

We know you'll be very happy to find a prone pose that you can still do! Poses like sphinx can be done with a bolster or blanket roll under your thighs. You can explore blocks under your hands or forearms, too. The goal is to feel a sense of lengthening and opening in the front of your body without feeling like there is uncomfortable compression in your lower back.

Inversions (headstands)

As we stated before, inversions are considered a possible issue because of the common shifts in balance during pregnancy. Going into a handstand or headstand can be very different now than it was a few weeks or months ago. That said, we were both practicing inversions well into our third trimesters, and so are many other yogis. As with standing balance poses, we'd recommend being closer to a wall if you normally practice in the middle of the room, so that you'll have support if you need it.

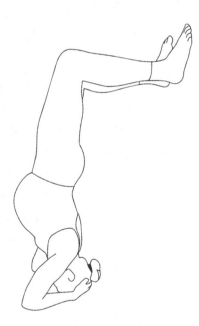

REFLECT
mindfulness and staying present

During the second trimester, it can often feel like one big waiting game. While this is often the most easeful trimester physically, it can be challenging to stay present. Because of increased energy and the recognition that this pregnancy is actually, really-and-truly happening, it can feel like there is so much to be done and so much anticipation of what is to come. Practicing mindfulness at this stage of pregnancy can be a useful tool to integrate awareness and acceptance of what is actually happening.

pregnancy

Felice Reddy, PhD, a clinical psychologist specializing in perinatal mental health, has this to say about practicing present-moment awareness during this time of great change:

In mindfulness, we are working to find ourselves again in this new territory. Mindfulness includes noticing, without judgment, the present moment—the physical sensations and the situation as it is without attaching our stories, fears, and judgments. We can start this work by thinking about our mind-body connection and building awareness of where we tend to feel tension and negative emotions in the body. Without trying to change them or wonder "why" they are here (whether it's pain, discomfort, or anxiety), we can let them be and notice: How does it feel, where does it show up, can I let it stay and also be present in the moment? This skill we practice on the mat translates directly to when we need to be present and calm in the middle of the night with a screaming baby or three years down the road with a tantrum over the wrong color spoon.

In mindfulness, we are working to find ourselves again in this new territory.

To engage with this practice of physical awareness and sensation, set aside ten minutes and take a comfortable seat or lie down. Starting at the very top of your head, move your awareness down the length of your body, pausing to notice sensation in each area of your body as your awareness rests there for a few breaths. Often, we are most aware of sensation in parts of our body that are feeling tight or tense or are experiencing some other uncomfortable sensation. Challenge yourself to pause for just as long a time at points that aren't experiencing as noticeable a sensation. See if you can fill up the entire ten minutes with this reflection and mindfulness exercise.

If you only have a few minutes, or even find yourself with a moment or two, notice what's happening. Can you feel your hands on the steering wheel? Are you aware of the cup of coffee or tea in your hand? How does the pillow feel against your head? Can you feel your feet firmly connect with the floor?

BREATHE
breath ratios: how to breathe when you're out of breath

You may notice that during the second trimester it gets a little harder to breathe. Partly, you may be more congested but, also, your rising uterus (and growing baby) is taking up more space. During her second pregnancy, Lauren wondered why her family had chosen to move into a home with a second floor before her daughter's arrival. Inhaling deeply and walking upstairs felt impossible. Good news: this next breath practice asks you to focus on your exhalation.

We breathe about 20,000 times a day, most of the time involuntarily. This practice gives you a chance to catch up with your breath. Breath ratios involve lengthening one part of your breath in relation to the other part. For this exercise, you'll lengthen your exhalation relative to your inhalation. Start by maybe a count of two more seconds and see how that feels. If it feels good to breathe out for even longer, you can lengthen your exhalation further. Keep in mind, you're not holding your breath on either side of the inhale or exhale: you're simply breathing out for longer.

To begin, get comfortable in any position and close your eyes if you'd like. As you inhale, count slowly in your mind to the number four. As you exhale, slow your breath and try to extend the exhalation to a count of six. If it feels like you're forcing this or running out of air to breathe out, shorten the ratio; try inhaling for four and exhaling for five. Conversely, if it takes you longer than a count of six to fully expel your breath, you could extend the ratio.

MOVE
hips and hamstrings sequence

The lower body needs a lot of love during pregnancy. The increased weight of your upper body places increased strain on your hips, pelvis, legs, and feet. Your pelvis may be less stable, leading to decreased stability in your hips. Side sleeping can add to the strain on the hips, and achiness is not uncommon during the second trimester of

pregnancy

pregnancy. Additionally, your growing belly can make it much more challenging to do any sort of forward folding, leading to increased tightness in the hamstrings and, as a result, the lower back. The following sequence will provide some relief for your hips and allow your hamstrings a little more movement and length. Having two blocks or the equivalent will be helpful for the poses below.

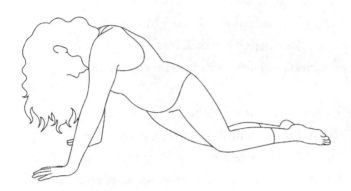

Hips side to side

Come to a tabletop position on your mat, with your knees under your hips and your hands under your shoulders. Allow your hips to sway from one side to the other—feel free to linger on either side if the outside stretch feels good.

Low lunge

From tabletop position, walk your hands over to the left, and bring your right foot forward. Keeping your front knee directly over (or slightly behind) your front foot, press your back knee down into the mat and energetically draw your front foot and your back knee toward each other, helping to stabilize the muscles in your hips and pelvis. You might place your hands on blocks on the inside of your front foot for more room for your belly.

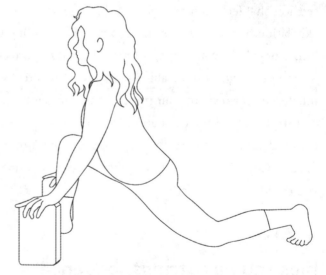

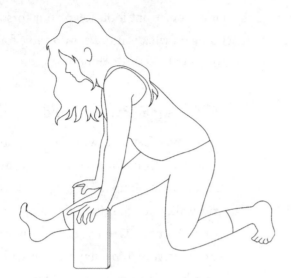

Runner's stretch

Keeping your front foot where it is, shift your hips back so they are directly over your back knee. Press your right heel into the floor and, without moving it, pull it back toward your hips. Use blocks on either side of your front leg, or on the inside of your front leg to create the length you need in this pose.

pregnancy

Open knee to side

Shift your hips forward again to come back into a lunge position with your right knee over your ankle. Begin to open your right knee out to the side, keeping your right foot active and flexed as you do this. Open your knee as far to the right as you'd like and as far as it feels good for your hip. This is one of Lauren's favorite poses and for years we've joked that she can't teach it without moaning with the joy of how good it feels!

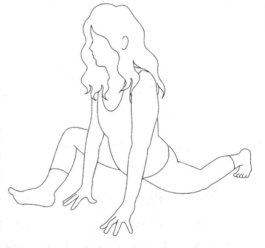

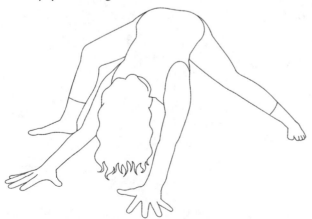

Side angle with hands and arms to inside

Lower the sole of your right foot back to the ground and lift your left knee off the floor. Drop the sole of your left foot to the floor, with the back edge of your foot either parallel to the back edge of your mat or angled slightly inward, coming into a Warrior 2 position with your legs. Walk your hands to the left of your front foot. Keep your torso elevated, or lower your front body more toward the floor, depending on what is more comfortable for you. Send your hips back in space and extend from your pelvis out and long through both legs.

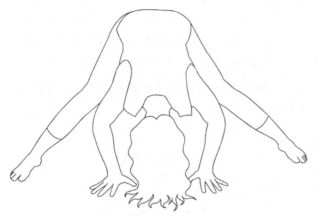

Wide-legged forward fold

Keep your feet in a wide stance and turn your front foot parallel to your back foot. Straighten both legs and, as you walk your hands to the space in front of and between your legs, make sure that your hips stay in line with your feet. How deeply you fold is up to you—use blocks under your hands to give yourself enough space and shorten the distance between your legs if a wider stance feels unstable or like it is too much.

Repeat the sequence on the second side.

Three-legged downward-facing dog

After you've completed the above sequence on the other side, step back into downward-facing dog, sweeping your right leg back and up. Bend your right knee and allow your foot to drop over to the left. If it feels good, add in a few hip circles or ankle rolls.

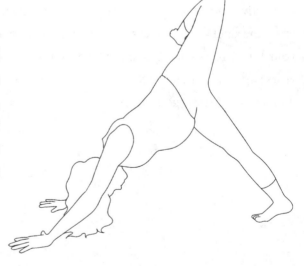

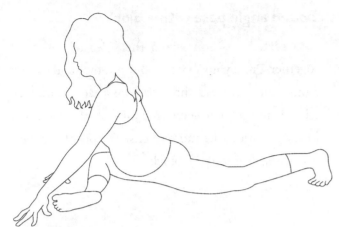

Pigeon pose

Sweep your right leg forward, bend your knee, and place your knee toward the right, upper corner of your mat. Your right foot can settle closer to your groin or closer to your left hand. Draw your left hip slightly forward and your right hip slightly back so your hips are fairly even with each other.

Repeat three-legged downward dog and pigeon pose on the other side.

Baby cradle pose

Come to sit in a cross-legged position. Pick up your right shin and calf and hold onto your lower leg with both hands. Rock your leg from side to side, stopping to explore any pockets of tightness or tension you feel in your outer hip.

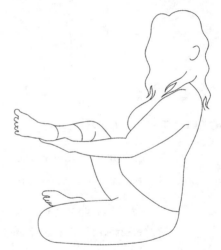

Firelog pose

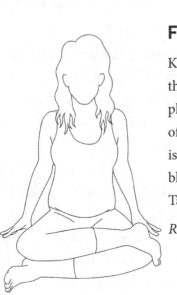

Keep your left shin parallel to the front edge of your mat and place your right ankle on top of your left knee, and your right knee on top of your left ankle. If there is a lot of space between your right knee and your left ankle, place a block or rolled up blanket there to support your knee and outer hip. Take several breaths here.

Repeat baby cradle and firelog pose on the other side.

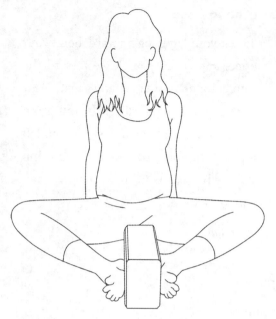

Bound angle pose with a block

In a seated position, bring the soles of your feet together. Press your feet into one another and extend from your pelvis out through both knees. Now, take a block and place it between your feet (the wider the block's position, the more intense the pose). Actively press your feet into the block.

RELATE
setting up to let go

Abigail, mother to two boys, ages five and three, shares how letting go was an important takeaway from her prenatal days.

There's the setting of intentions, and then there's the letting go. I learned this lesson each week as I felt how my body had changed from the week prior and discovered that what felt good then might feel very different now. Savasana now required bolsters and pillows. Sometimes I would enter the yoga studio flush with energy, only to find that resting in child's pose felt best—the intention and the letting go.

I learned that lesson most deeply during my birth—an unexpected surgical birth, a loss of control, a postpartum period that went in exactly the opposite way that I had intended. The breath work helped. All those squats helped. But the most meaningful by far, the place I kept returning to, was the practice of letting go. Could I release my disappointment in myself, just as I'm reminded on the mat to release the tension in my face? Could I let go of an intention that did not materialize, and find peace in what took its place?

I think we forget too easily that birth is a psychological transformation as much as a physical one. My yoga practice during pregnancy gave me a way to connect with my changing body, but even more important was the perspective it gave me on my own expectations of that body. The hope for a certain kind of experience, and the reality that takes its place: the intention, the letting go, and the beauty in both.

WISDOM
Kegels, schmegels: pelvic floor and vaginal birth

There are a lot of articles to be found about the importance of doing Kegels during pregnancy. (You can practice them in line at the grocery store! To engage these muscles, pretend that you're stopping the flow of urine! Three cheers for Kegels!) In all seriousness, while strong pelvic floor muscles can be useful in reducing the chance of incontinence and a sense of heaviness in the pelvis both during and after pregnancy, and for birth, these muscles don't need to be toned, tight, and strong. In fact, their biggest role during birth is to move the heck out of the way to allow room for the baby to pass through on their way out of the vaginal canal. The uterus and muscles of the abdomen, along with pressure within the abdomen, are what are crucial to push the baby out.

Certified Nurse Midwife Meg Berreth told us that she tells her patients that they should strive to have a "body builder's arms, a marathon runner's legs, and a couch potato's pelvic floor." So, rather than strength, it is flexibility and the ability to relax on demand that will allow the muscles of the pelvic floor to stretch—two to three times their original length (!) and space in order to make room for your baby's head to emerge. Especially if this is your first birth experience, it is more likely that you have tight or hypertonic pelvic floor muscles rather than overly lax muscles. The most important thing you can do for the muscles of your pelvic floor is to work with exercises that help relax them. After gaining good control of the relaxation response in the pelvic floor, you can work to alternately strengthen and relax the same muscles, which will be most helpful for you during pregnancy and after delivery. The most helpful exercise for connecting with and relaxing the muscles deep in your pelvic bowl is diaphragmatic breathing, which we explain next.

pregnancy

BREATHE
how do you breathe? diaphragmatic breathing

Diaphragmatic breathing, also sometimes called belly breathing, is a breath practice that shows up in some of the other types of pranayama that we mention in this book. Diaphragmatic breathing can help you feel more relaxed, and some research suggests that it increases how much oxygen is in your blood and reduces your heart rate. Diaphragmatic breathing is the ideal way to breathe, but sometimes stress or changes in your weight or posture (ahem, pregnancy), can cause your breathing to become shallower.

When you inhale, here's what happens in your body: Your lungs and chest expand, your rib cage moves both upward and outward, and your diaphragm contracts, flattens, and moves downward in your body. The space that your diaphragm vacates is filled by your expanded lungs. When you exhale, your lungs and chest relax, reducing the space in your chest, and your lungs deflate. Your diaphragm relaxes, lifts, and returns to its (original) dome-like shape.

To practice diaphragmatic breathing, sit or lie back so that you can prop your hands on your belly. Relax your shoulders, your face, your neck, your jaw. If possible, inhale and exhale through your nose. As you inhale, notice your belly expanding outward. Notice the sensation of full expansion in your lungs. As you exhale, feel your belly soften and notice the effortlessness at the bottom of your breath out before you inhale again. Try to keep your shoulders in the same position throughout, focusing the movement of this breath on your belly and chest.

MOVE
connect to your pelvic floor

Connecting to your pelvic floor while you're pregnant requires an awareness of the muscles in the pelvic floor space and being able to soften them, release them, and relax them. This ability to release is crucial to labor and delivery. Kelly Raney, CFm, PRPC, COMT, Cert. DN, pelvic floor physical therapist, notes that "Pushing out a baby requires abdominal activation. This strength is needed to create pressure, along with uterine contractions, to help your baby descend into the birth canal. From there, the pelvic floor muscles have to expand to allow passage through the canal."

For these two pelvic floor poses, there isn't much movement: Come into the pose and hang there. In both shapes, you get a chance to practice deep diaphragmatic breathing and to focus on relaxing your pelvic floor muscles as you breathe in. You'll want two blocks and a bolster or couch cushion for these poses.

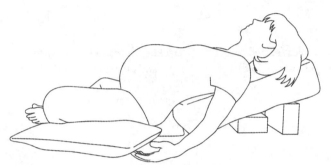

Reclined bound angle

Create a ramp with your blocks and bolster or couch cushion, so you can recline back, keeping your head above your heart. Bring the soles of your feet together and allow your knees to drop out to the sides. (Your heels can be as close or far from your groin as is comfortable.) You might bring your hands to your belly as a helpful reminder to keep your breath rooted in that space. As you inhale, do so fully, allowing your lungs and belly to rise and fill. If you'd like, you can lightly contract your pelvic floor on the exhalation—think of it as a baby Kegel. As you inhale, release your belly and pelvic floor. Some imagery may be helpful here: As you breathe in, imagine the bones at the bottom of your pelvis (commonly called sitting bones, anatomically called *ischial tuberosities*) spreading wider apart. Take between five to ten breaths focused on your diaphragmatic breathing and pelvic floor musculature release, and rest here as long as you'd like.

Supported low squat

Have a seat on a bolster or one or two blocks. Sit in a squatting position and bring your hands to your thighs or your heart center. If you do the latter, you can even use your elbows to create gentle resistance against your legs. In this position, again bring your attention to your pelvic floor and your breath: As you exhale, do so completely with a light contraction of your pelvic floor. As you inhale, do so completely, keeping your focus on fully releasing and softening your pelvic floor.

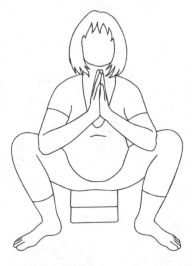

common modifications for your practice

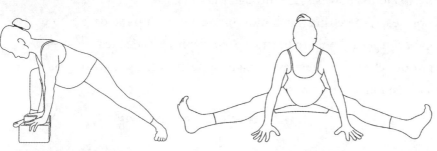

Standing poses (humble warrior)

Forward folds (seated
wide-legged forward fold)

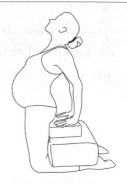

Backbends (camel with bolster
and blocks on calves)

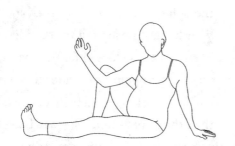

Twisting (open twist in half
lord of the fishes pose)

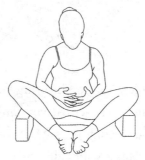

Seated hip openers (seated bound angle
on cushion, block under each knee)

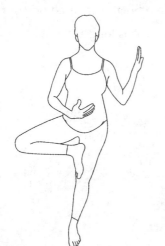

Balancing poses (tree at wall)

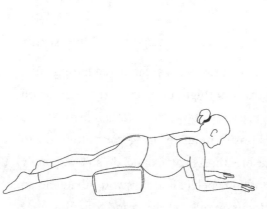

Belly-down poses
(sphinx with bolster under hips)

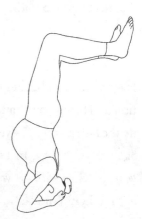

Inversions (headstands)

hips and hamstrings sequence

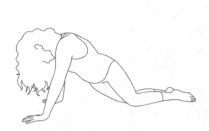

Hips side to side

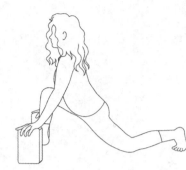

Low lunge

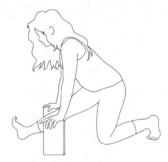

Runner's stretch

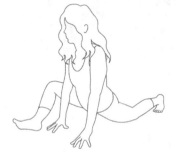

Open knee to side

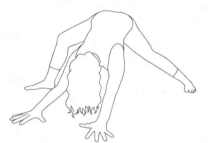

Side angle with hands and
arms to inside

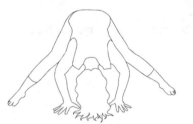

Wide-legged forward fold

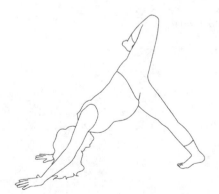

Three-legged downward-facing dog

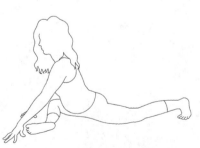

Pigeon pose

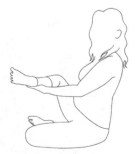

Baby cradle pose

pregnancy

hips and hamstrings sequence (continued)

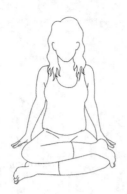

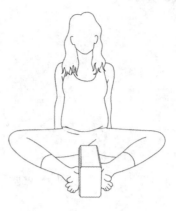

Firelog pose

Bound angle pose with a block

connect to your pelvic floor

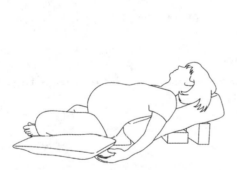

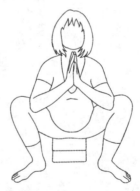

Reclined bound angle

Supported low squat

Chapter Five

trimester three: it's scientifically impossible to be ninety weeks pregnant

You're close to the finish line—it's in sight. What are you more excited for at this moment? Meeting your baby? Tying your own shoes? The cessation of heartburn? If pregnancy is a road race, you're in the last mile. You can see that there is indeed a stopping point (though it may feel elusive and surreal at times). And sometimes that casts the entire race in a more pleasant light. Trimester three is the last period of enjoying having your baby tucked away, of enjoying a quieter household, of enjoying the experience of pregnancy (and if it's your first child, the experience of pregnancy *without* the experience of parenting). Sometimes the opposite feels true. There is trepidation and excitement regarding what is to come, whether this is your first or fifth baby.

Let's start with this chapter's title: It is happily unlikely that you will make it to ninety weeks pregnant. Depending on your choices and your doctor or midwife's thoughts, you may make it past forty weeks, though. According to the data-driven online childbirth resource, *Evidence-Based Birth*, "About half of all pregnant people will go into labor on their own by forty weeks and five days (for first-time mothers) or forty weeks and three days (for mothers who have given birth before). The other half will not." So, you have a good chance of walking past your due date with strangers still asking when your baby is arriving.

How do you feel this trimester? You might feel extremely tired. You might feel like the body you are moving, breathing, and sleeping in (or trying to sleep in) is very unfamiliar and very much not your own. Pregnancy is an alien landscape (with an alien invader!) and it's really okay if you don't love this part. Or maybe you *do* love this part, with the attendant sweetness of baby kicks and the omnipresence of your little one's movement. Whether you feel icky or lovely, you get to feel exactly how you feel: no apology or explanation needed.

Anecdotally, women sometimes report feeling bouts of big energy and a laser-sharp focus on organizing and getting their home ready for the new arrival. That makes sense; when there is so much we can't control, putting our energy into what we *can* control often imbues us with an overall sense of empowerment. Do what you need to feel safe, empowered, and on top of things. In addition to home organization and traditional "nesting," some other ways to handle all the big feelings of impending change and anticipation are to practice meditation, use mantra, and explore your breath. Since the last trimester of pregnancy is about big changes, in this chapter we'll explore reflections to that end. We remember those days of huffing and puffing up even the tiniest hill, so we'll look at breathing practices that can help when you're experiencing *dyspnea* (shortness of breath), provide you with mantras to help when you're feeling impatient, yogic philosophy to guide your final weeks, and movement to help you when moving is the very, very, very last thing you feel like doing.

WISDOM
and *now*? what's happening in my body *now*?

In the third trimester (weeks 28–40+), there may be a lot of physical sensations that were not part of the previous trimesters. By about week thirty-five, your uterus is just below your breastbone and ribs. Your uterus is also practicing its eventual work, like a runner doing laps before a marathon, and while you may or may not feel your Braxton-Hicks contractions, you are definitely having them.

In addition to growing a baby, you've also been growing an entire organ: At full term, your baby's placenta is six-to-eight inches in diameter and one-inch thick. It weighs about a pound!

Leading into birth, your baby might be lightening (dropping) into your pelvis. Your cervix may begin softening and effacing (thinning), and the amniotic fluid surrounding your baby may be decreasing. Your joints might feel looser than ever, as your body weight grows, and hormones continue their good work of preparing your pelvis for delivery.

During this final trimester, you may experience heartburn. (Alexandra recently taught a prenatal yoga class where a student showed up and placed a bottle of Tums at the top of her mat. When others noticed, she offered them out like breath mints!) Indigestion and constipation may be companions of this period, too.

As your baby grows and your uterus expands, your diaphragm and internal organs get a little smooshed. As a result, you might feel even more short of breath. The weight of your baby, uterus, placenta, amniotic fluid (and on and on) on your bladder might mean you need to pee even more frequently now, and sleep may be more challenging as a result. Sleep can also be affected because of the discomfort of being in a body so very different from the one you inhabited nine months ago, and the increased need to change positions in the middle of the night.

At this point, it almost feels silly to go over even more possible pregnancy complaints. We've joked in our prenatal classes that we should print T-shirts that say, "My back hurts, I haven't slept in weeks, I have constant heartburn, my belly itches, I am hot all the time, and *everything* is swollen. But, other than that, I'm great!" The end of pregnancy is generally not incredibly comfortable and, in addition to the other challenges mentioned, you may also experience numbness or tingling in your hands, swelling in your legs and feet, abdominal itching as your skin expands, changes in balance, production of colostrum, hemorrhoids, varicose veins, and sharp zings of nerve pain in your nether region—typically called "lightning crotch." The fun never ends!

But, actually, it will, and likely sooner than you can imagine.

pregnancy

special considerations

It is in the third trimester when your yoga practice is most likely to need some adjustments. It will probably feel more comfortable in your body to slightly shift the way you have typically practiced. The third trimester is also a time when certain pregnancy-related issues might arise. Fortunately, sometimes small shifts can be helpful in mitigating whatever physical challenge you're facing.

Problems with carpal tunnel, and similarly presenting wrist and hand pain and numbness, are more likely to occur during the third trimester because of the increase of fluid in the body and resulting pressure on the ulnar and median nerves in the wrist. To counter wrist pressure in many yoga poses, consider purchasing a wrist wedge or rolling up the front of your mat to create a ramp for your hands. Alternatively, you can lower to your forearms on blocks or on the floor.

If your baby is presenting as breech after the thirty-second week of pregnancy, we recommend avoiding deep squatting positions, or other poses that open the pelvis and place direct pressure on the cervical outlet. Although a different issue entirely, pubic bone pain caused by *pubic symphysis dysfunction* (or even just an abundance of pelvic pressure) can be helped by avoiding wide-legged positions, and omitting poses that open your legs away from each other.

Due to a confluence of factors, heartburn often looms large in the third trimester. While there isn't a specific pose or set of poses that can be particularly helpful in mitigating it, poses that require the head to be below the heart and belly (standing forward fold or downward-facing dog, for example), can exacerbate the issue. Be sure to have blocks, or something similar, available as you practice in order to keep your head parallel to your heart and not lower.

Sciatic nerve pain—which can feel like radiating pain from your hip to or toward your knee—is another common consideration that can often flare in the third trimester, though other trimesters are not immune. Sciatic nerve pain in pregnancy is most often caused by the swelling of the *piriformis* (a deep gluteal muscle) that then presses against the sciatic nerve, causing pain. Alternating between deep gluteal stretches (like figure-four stretch and variations on pigeon) and engagement of the muscles of your seat (in poses like squat or bridge) can be a useful way to relieve the discomfort of pregnancy-related sciatica.

MOVE
sequence for creating space

When your body is growing bigger and bigger by the day, it feels impossible to create any room between your hips and your ribs: Instead, your cozy little roommate is nestled in there, and it may feel next to impossible to just lengthen out. This sequence will help you feel a little more spacious and open. Using a wall for this sequence may be helpful. A bolster or pillow will be useful, too.

Sit cozy against a wall

Begin seated on the floor on a mat, against the wall, with a bolster or pillow supporting your seat and lower back. Take several rounds of breath, working to lift your sternum away from your belly and breathe into the sides of your waist, paying particular attention to the back of your body.

Seated side stretch

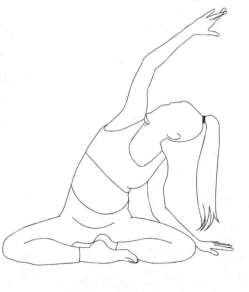

Come fully upright, in a cross-legged position, and place your left hand to the left of your body, pressing into the floor, and bending your arm at the elbow. Stretch your right arm up and over the right side of your face and take a deep, full breath into the right side of your waist, picturing your lower ribs untethering themselves from your right-side waist. Take a few full breaths and repeat on the other side.

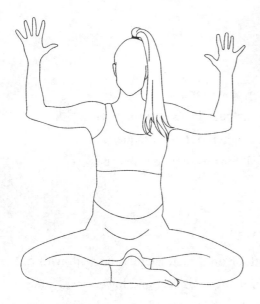

Cactus-arms seat

In the same cross-legged position, bring both arms out to the side and bend them at the elbow, working to bring your elbow, forearm, and upper arm behind the front plane of your chest. Either remain in this static position for a few breaths or alternate between having your arms bent at your side and stretching them up overhead.

Open-hearted seat

Bring your hands behind your lower back and interlace your fingers. Bend your elbows such that you can place your knuckles at the small of your back to gently press into your sacrum. Manually, and gently, extend your lower back (both physically and mentally) toward the ground. Keep your head in line with your spine and draw your baby energetically toward the back plane of your body.

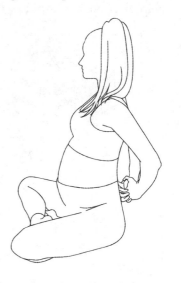

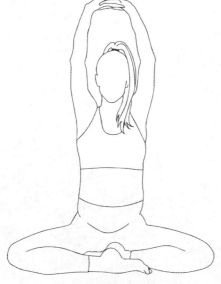

Sky-reach seat

Slowly begin to straighten your arms and extend your interlaced hands upward. After a few breaths, release your hands and take a moment to check in with your front body, again picturing the creation of space between your sternum and your baby and belly.

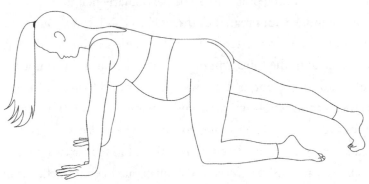

Tabletop calf stretch

Come on to your hands and knees, with your knees under your hips and your hands under your shoulders. Extend your right leg behind you, with the toes of your right foot tucked under, on the floor. Stretch back through your right calf.

Knee-down, side angle stretch

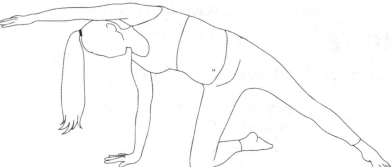

Lower your right foot to the floor, so that the outer edge of your foot is parallel to the back edge of your mat. With your left knee still on the floor, you may choose to angle your shin away from your body to provide a better base of support and make it easier to balance. Extend your right arm alongside your right ear. Picture your breath moving into the space of your side body, making room and creating length.

After a few breaths, transition back to tabletop position and repeat the last two movements on the other side.

BREATHE
bee breath

To practice *brahmari pranayama* (bee breath), sit comfortably with your shoulders relaxed. Start by taking a few natural breaths and close your eyes. Then, keeping the lips lightly sealed, inhale through the nostrils. Exhaling, make the sound of the letter M or the sound of the letters N and G together—essentially a humming sound. Sustain the sound until you need to inhale. Then repeat: Inhale through the nose, then hum like a buzzing bee as you exhale. Continue by inhaling as needed and exhaling with this sound for several minutes. This breathing practice can be particularly helpful if you feel your anxiety amping up as the end of your pregnancy draws closer, as it gives your mind something audible on which to focus your attention. For the same reason, in addition to being a helpful breath practice in the third trimester, brahmari can be a wonderful pranayama practice to utilize during labor as it allows your mind to focus on the audible quality of your breath. As contractions increase and sensations in your body grow more intense, bee breath can offer a respite by giving you somewhere else to focus your effort and attention. It's also pleasant to practice this breath in tandem with someone else (or many other people), so that the buzzing sounds you create become a chorus or tonal backdrop to your birth experience.

MOVE
sequence for lower-back love

Low-back pain during pregnancy is common because as your belly grows, your posture shifts, and your lower-back muscles are asked to work harder. In addition, your joints and ligaments are preparing for birth and labor, loosening as a result. The sacro-iliac joints (SI joints) connect the pelvis and lower spine, and we often hear about the one-sided pain that joint discomfort can cause. Because of the instability of the low back and all the asymmetrical movement necessary for life, one-sided lower back pain is common. Stability is key for the SI joints of the low back. If discomfort is flaring on one side or the other, work with symmetry in movement as much as possible. If your complaint is general achiness, try the following sequence to give your lower back some time and attention. To practice the following poses, it's helpful to be set up close to a wall and to have blocks to use.

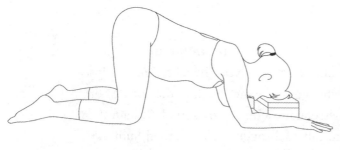

Modified puppy pose

Come to all fours on your mat. Keeping your hips over your knees, lower to your forearms and place a block under your forehead for support. You can remain still or rock your hips a bit from side to side, directing your breath into the back plane of your body.

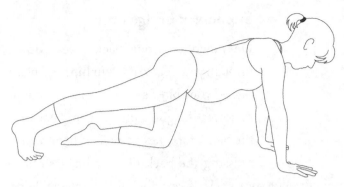

Tabletop with leg cross

From puppy pose, come back up to your hands and knees and stretch your right leg long, keeping your toes tucked under and your foot on the floor. Then, slowly lift your leg, maintaining the space in your low back as you do so, and cross your right leg over the calf of your left leg, once again lowering the toes of your right foot to the floor. Press back through your inner heel and turn your gaze over your left shoulder. After coming back to center, repeat this on your left side.

Downward-facing dog

From all fours, tuck your toes under and lift your knees, coming into downward-facing dog. You might bend one knee and then the other or try swaying your hips here. Take time to listen to your lower back, and move around in ways that help it feel looser and free.

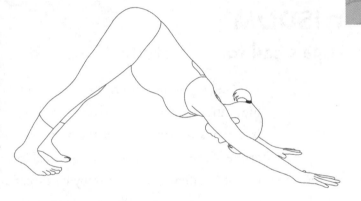

Supported squat at the wall

From down dog, walk your hands back to your feet. Place a block or two in front of the wall. Take a seat on the support of the block(s). With your feet on the ground, knees bent, lean your back body against the wall and lift up through your sternum as you sink more heavily into the support of the block(s).

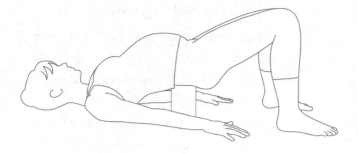

Supported bridge pose

Lie down on your back. Press down through your feet to lift your hips and place one of your blocks under your sacrum at its lowest height. Rest your low back on the block for a few rounds of breath, also pressing the back of your head straight down into the ground to maintain the natural curve of your neck. If you don't feel comfortable on your back for even a short period of time, omit this pose.

WISDOM
yoga's call for self-study

One joy of the third trimester is that you have a chance to reflect on what you want life in the postpartum era to bring while your baby is still being cared for and comforted in a hands-off way. In yoga, the word *svadhayaya* means to study yourself. Svadhayaya is one of the niyamas, or the healthy habits that are a part of the yogic path. Svadhayaya is a little different from therapy or psychoanalysis. It's more akin to something more ethereal and spiritual, like "knowing your own essence." So how do you study yourself? Much of the other suggestions in this chapter are part of self-study: When you take time to be alone, move, breathe, and reflect, you're doing the work to know yourself. More active reflection and journaling are helpful, too.

Using this time period of your pregnancy to consider who you are, what sort of mother or parent you want to be, and what you want your motherhood or parenthood life to look like can be part of svadhayaya. Creating space for this self-reflection (and self-study) may mean a smoother entry (or reentry) into the early days of being a care-giver. One way to reflect and prepare for what's to come is by asking yourself questions about your ideal scenarios for your future life with your baby. If you have a partner or other support person in this journey, it's equally important that they clearly articulate their needs and expectations as the two (three) of you embark on this journey.

MOVE
sequence for edema

We know, we know: You're puffy. Your hands are puffy. Your feet are puffy. One of the downsides of pregnancy is all the swelling. Once, after walking around an IKEA all day while pregnant, Alexandra's husband made a joke about the size of her swollen ankles. (Don't worry; she got the last laugh. Who do you think put all the new furniture together? Not the woman with the engorged feet, that's for sure.) During pregnancy, your body is holding more fluid than usual. If the weather is hot or you've had to sit or stand for a longer period of time, that fluid can gather in your legs, feet, and ankles. This sequence won't solve it, but it can help. For this sequence, you may want two blocks and a bolster or couch cushion. You'll need to set up near a wall. (And you can even do this sequence in bed, using the wall at the head of your bed as the rest for your legs.)

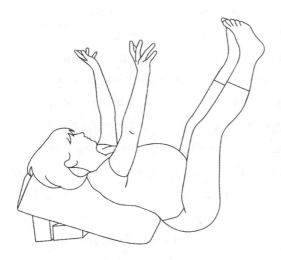

Supported fish pose with wall support

Set up a supported pose by draping your body over a bolster (or couch cushion) that is raised higher at one end. (You can place the cushion or bolster on a block or stack of books to angle it.) Position your sitting bones between the bolster setup and the wall and slide your legs up the wall. If the space between your bolster and the wall is smaller, the angle and positioning of your legs will be greater. Stay here, allowing your legs to temporarily change their relationship to gravity and hopefully provide a little relief from swelling. If you are also having issues with swelling or tingling in your hands, reach your arms overhead and alternate between making a tight fist and uncurling your fingers.

REFLECT
let go

When Alexandra was in her thirty-sixth or thirty-seventh week of pregnancy, she declared to a friend: "I've figured out the secret to pregnancy! It's about letting go of having control." Her friend—a mother of two—smiled slightly and said, "Ah, but you've actually figured out the secret to parenthood, too." So much of being pregnant is about letting go of (more accurately, the illusion of) control. Your body changes quickly in an extreme way, and there's little you can do but hang on for the ride (and try to sleep). Motherhood brings this same challenge: quick adaptation to rapid changes.

It's about letting go of having control.

If you're pregnant for the first time, the joy of the third trimester is that you still have a little more alone time. If you're already mothering-in-action, meditation and reflection can be harder to fit in. Regardless of whether you have twenty minutes or two minutes, here's a meditation practice to explore.

It's helpful, if possible, to practice this meditation in a space where you are completely physically supported. Then, start by identifying your feet. You can move them, flex them, or wiggle them. Take a full breath in, and, as you exhale, relax your feet completely, and allow them to come to stillness. As this occurs, you might think to yourself, *Let go*. Next, focus on your calves and ankles. You might squeeze the muscles of your calves onto the bones as you inhale. As you exhale, fully release those muscles, and think again: *Let go*. Continue this exploration of light engagement and movement of each part of your body on the inhale and then full relaxation on your exhale. Each time you exhale and release a part of your body, give yourself permission to let go. Move through your hips and seat, your belly space, your ribs and chest, your shoulders, your upper arms, your forearms, your hands. Then bring that same attention of gentle engagement and full relaxation to your neck, jaw, mouth, lips, cheeks, nose, eyes, eyebrows, forehead, ears, and skull.

Once you've completed this meditation practice of moving through your body and letting go, you might just lie still and breathe for a while, with no agenda except to marinate in the sweetness of having let it all go.

MOVE
yoga for winding down for good sleep

We know how elusive sleep can be throughout pregnancy, and particularly in the third trimester. The following movements can serve as a nice ritual before bed and can set you up to be as relaxed as possible before you try to catch those evasive ZZZs.

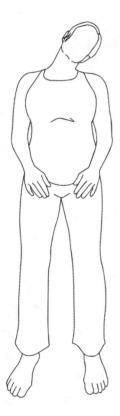

Neck rolls

Come to any kind of seat that feels comfortable to you and allow your chin to drop toward your chest. Keeping your movement slow, allow your chin to trace a half or third of a circle across the front of your chest. If it feels good to drop your right ear toward your right shoulder and your left ear toward your left shoulder, please do.

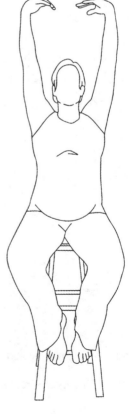

Wrist rolls

Move your hands around in circles, either keeping them in one place, or moving them as you lift and lower your arms in rhythm with your breath.

pregnancy

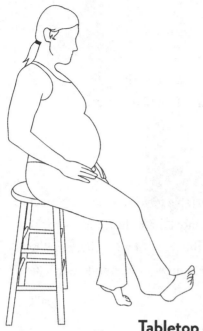

Ankle rolls

Whether sitting on a chair or on the ground, extend your legs long and point and flex your feet. Circle your feet around, exploring the fullest range of movement and stretching out through your toes as well as your feet.

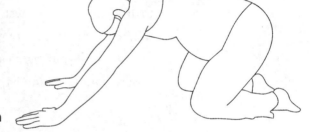

Tabletop exploration

Come up to your hands and knees. Close your eyes if it feels okay to do so and begin to move in any intuitive way that feels good. This movement could involve hip circles or swaying from side to side or any variation of cat/dog.

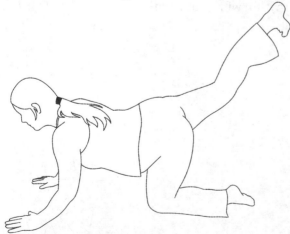

Tiger stretch

Remaining in tabletop position, extend your right leg straight back. Tuck your toes under and pulse back a few times through your heel. Slowly begin to lift your leg, keeping your lower back long and your tailbone extending toward your heel. If you're able to maintain the length in your lower back, you might even elevate your leg higher than the level of your hip, drawing your sternum forward and gazing up as you stretch out from your pelvis in both directions.

Repeat this tiger stretch on the other side.

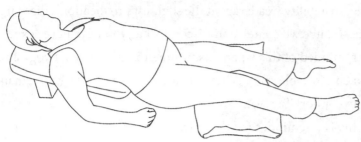

Tense and release

You can be seated, standing, or supine for this exercise. Begin by slowly counting to ten and, as you do, start to tense as many parts of your body as you are able. Purse your lips, wrinkle your nose, make fists with your hands, clench your jaw, and tighten the muscles of your arms and legs. Hold for a beat or two when you reach ten, and then slowly begin to release the tension throughout your body.

Legs up the wall

Set up a ramp of support a foot and a half or two feet away from a wall, using a bolster and a few blocks, or anything else that forms a comfortable, elevated support for your upper body. Bring your seat in front of your bolster and scoot your legs up the wall. If you need more space, move your setup farther away from the wall. Conversely, if you want to elevate your legs more, bring your setup closer to the wall.

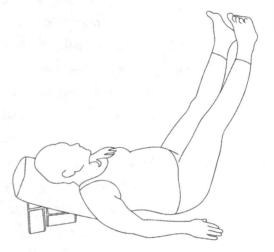

RELATE
"take a comfortable seat": waiting for your baby to arrive

Lauren offers solid advice for the end of the third trimester, will-baby-ever-come? days:

I was pregnant for eighty-nine weeks with my daughter. Okay, forty-one weeks. However, if anyone is looking to slow time, just spend a week as a pregnant woman who has gone past her due date. It was the longest week of my life. Like the movie *Groundhog*

Day, except with swelling, irritability (read: rage at the slightest provocation), discharge from all manner of places (you're welcome), and discomfort as you have never experienced. Sometimes I am reminded of this when I ask women in my prenatal yoga class to "take a comfortable seat." When you are eighty-nine weeks pregnant, there is no comfortable seat.

When you are eighty-nine weeks pregnant, there is no comfortable seat.

So, this is a reminder for those women whose due date has come and gone, who have strangers tremble in fear at their approach, who have to tell the eighth person today that "No, I am not having twins." There is so much more that I wish I could offer. But, because I know that perusing websites for anything and everything to kickstart labor gets old, I will share my own to-do list. None of these suggestions will help you welcome your baby any more quickly. Nevertheless, I found several of them helpful during those final (and so, so long) days.

- Take baths. Long ones, with water that comes over your belly. Close your eyes and assure yourself that labor is definitely starting tonight.
- Alternatively, if it's 3,000 degrees out, find a pool. Buy twelve foam noodles at Target and use all of them.
- Punch your big pregnancy pillow.
- Play some mindless game on your phone, pausing only to film your alien belly as it morphs.
- Take pictures of your swollen legs and send them to your friends. Encourage them to feel really sorry for you.
- Cry. If you don't feel like crying, cry about that.
- Go to the grocery store (or send someone for you). Buy that food item that you never buy because there are too many calories and it's not sensible and you might feel judged at the checkout, and it won't taste as good as you remember it tasting. Cheers to another reason for feeling sorry for yourself.
- Strap a heating pad to some part of you that hurts. Move it when another part of you hurts.
- If you don't feel like lifting yourself up off the floor, do not do it.

- If you do feel like lifting yourself off the floor, get into hands and knees and round your back. Do cat like you've never done cat before. I also found that lowering onto my forearms and rocking back and forth (moaning optional) helped.
- If there are things that need to "get done" around the house, make sure that you are not the one "getting them done."
- If you have heartburn that rivals that of the winner of a chili-eating contest, crush a bunch of Tums on top of a huge bowl of ice cream in consolation.
- Daydream about when you'll be able to bend at the waist again.

I *promise* you won't make it to ninety weeks.

REFLECT
mantras for the end of pregnancy

As we've discussed in previous chapters, mantra is a powerful tool for intention-creating. We love the idea of using mantra to move our heads into the spaces we desire. You can use mantra as you drive, walk, when you wake up, or during meditation. Here are some suggested mantras for the third trimester of pregnancy. You can add mantra to a breath practice by inhaling for half the mantra and exhaling for the other half. (Or by "inhaling" your mantra and exhaling its opposite. Something like "Inhale, accepting; exhale, controlling" makes a nice mantra and breath practice.)

I'm ready for this change.
I'll meet my baby soon.
My heart and life are expanding.
I accept things as they are in this moment.
Heart open, mind steady.

sequence for creating space

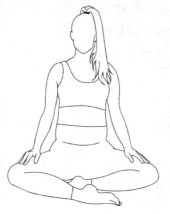

Sit cozy against a wall

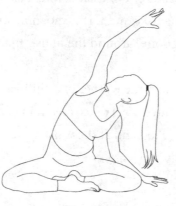

Seated side stretch

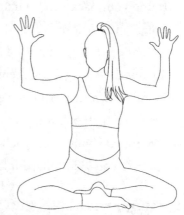

Cactus-arms seat

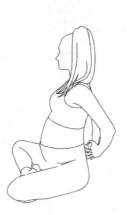

Open-hearted seat

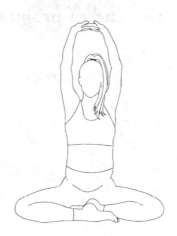

Sky-reach seat

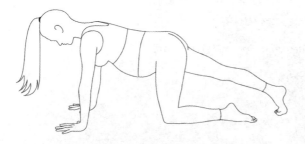

Tabletop calf stretch

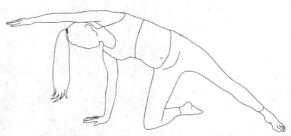

Knee-down, side angle stretch

sequence for lower-back love

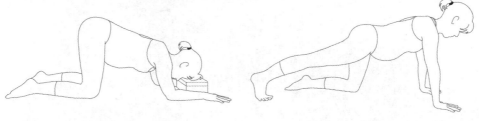

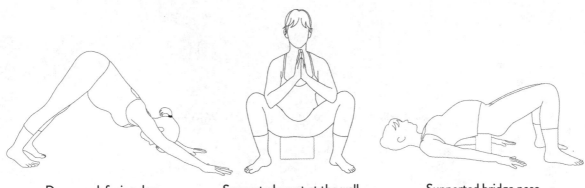

Modified puppy pose

Tabletop with leg cross

Downward-facing dog

Supported squat at the wall.

Supported bridge pose

sequence for edema

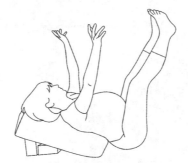

Supported fish pose with wall support

yoga for winding down for good sleep

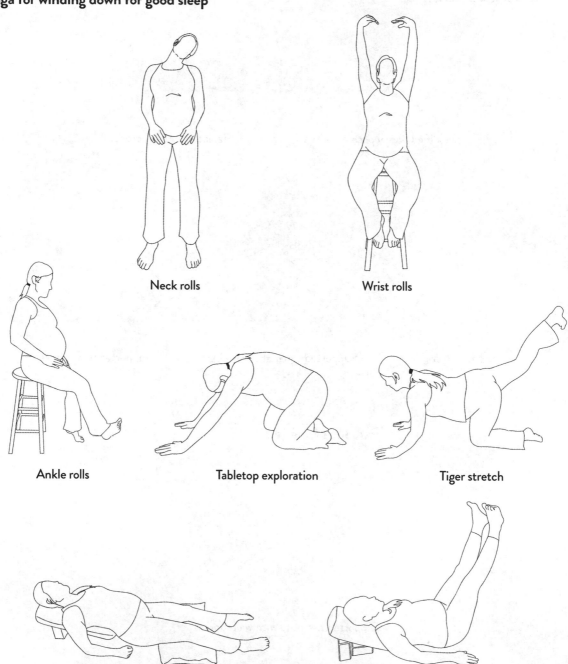

Neck rolls

Wrist rolls

Ankle rolls

Tabletop exploration

Tiger stretch

Tense and release

Legs up the wall

Part Three

labor and birth

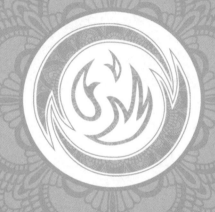

Chapter Six

yoga for the intensity of labor and birth

In prenatal yoga, it is sometimes assumed that there is a certain end-goal birth experience in mind—alternatively called "natural birth," "unmedicated birth," or "unassisted birth"—and that the practice of yoga will be fundamental in allowing you to achieve that goal. It's true that yoga will provide the tools and guidance to help you follow your breath, tune in to the present moment, and offer you more awareness of the needs and sensations occurring in your body. As we noted earlier in this book, it's even possible that yoga can speed up labor. We believe in the power of yoga as a movement modality and philosophical practice to offer support for birth and labor, and if you have a goal of an unmedicated birth, we know that the tools of yoga will be of service to you and that your yoga practice will play an important role in preparing you to weather the sensations of contractions and the beauty and wildness of birth.

But no yoga pose will shift your pubic bone or change the size and shape of your baby's head. No breath practice will alter the capacity of your cervix to dilate. And in a majority of cases, if your baby is in a breech position, no number of bridge poses will cause your little one to do a uterine 180 (although there's probably no harm in trying!). In short, there are aspects of your birth experience that are within your control. And there may be aspects of your birth experience that are not. In either case, yoga can support you.

Historically, birth was an unmedicated, private home event. Through the 1900s, it transitioned to a pathologized, medicalized hospital event. Currently, the large majority of births in America take place in hospitals and are attended by doctors.

As a result, there has been obvious and necessary pushback. Over the past fifty years, there has been a rise in midwifery, doula use, and births at home or birth centers. That said, the percentage of out-of-hospital births in the United States is fewer than 2 percent. Nearly a third of all births in the United States are cesarean deliveries. Birth is still, by and large, treated as a medical event in need of a medical setting with medical intervention. (And sometimes *it is* a medical event, in need of a medical setting and medical intervention for the health and safety of the baby and birthing parent.)

Over the past fifty years, there has been a rise in midwifery, doula use, and births at home or birth centers.

We also want to acknowledge the paradox around cesarean births: the United States has a much higher rate than the current World Health Organization recommended rate of 10 percent or fewer births by cesarean. While all birth is birth, and we applaud the medical possibilities available to create safe birth options for all mothers, there is tremendous research that suggests that not all American cesarean births are medically necessary. It's no wonder, then, that there is a distrust of medicalizing birth.

The shift away from medicalized birth is a win for mothers and birthing people. Not many years ago, episiotomies (surgical cuts made around the vagina) were routine, as were narcotic substances that either anesthetized birthing people completely or made them very disconnected from the experience. And while many birthing people still lack control over their own birth choices (in part because of systemic racism or differences in care in relation to wealth), in many areas of the country, birth has become an experience in which women can feel empowered with good medical knowledge to make choices that feel intuitive and right for them. As yoga practitioners, we celebrate this.

But the pendulum swings a little wide sometimes, and as a result of this gentle return to a preference for unmedicated, natural birth, the need for medicalized birth (as in therapeutics to alleviate suffering, medications to speed up or slow down birth, and cesarean procedures to allow the baby or mother or both to stay safe) have become subtly demonized. Birth parents who desire pain support or need medical care have somehow become emblems of failure in certain pockets of American culture—the same pockets that often gravitate to yoga.

You may be coming into your birth with a list of hopes for the experience. You may have some very clear birth preferences. You've done your research and visualized what you want and what alternatives might occur. But no matter your preferences, hopes, or preparations, birth happens. Sometimes it happens with fairy lights and classical music and three pushes. Sometimes it comes after sixty hours of labor, when you've made it to 9 centimeters, and your care provider wheels you into a brightly lit operating room. It happens with medication and without, and sometimes babies come into this world via vaginal canal, and sometimes via an abdominal and uterine incision. (Although, as far as we know, never through your armpit, as Lauren's son once guessed about his sister's upcoming birth!)

In a birth setting, you have the right to autonomy over your body—to feel empowered to make the decisions that are best for you and your baby. The goal of a yoga practice during preconception and pregnancy is not to have a moonlit birth in a river, completely without assistance (although that does sound pretty lovely!). Instead, we want you to feel connected and in touch with your body, supported by your loved ones and care providers, and because of your innate knowledge, your intuition, and your birth team, you feel empowered to make the best decisions available to you at any given moment—whatever path your birth takes.

Yoga is about union—a yoking of body, mind, and spirit. Awareness and engagement with your body, mind, and spirit are paramount during labor, regardless of what that labor looks like. Yoga philosophy doesn't speculate on whether you get the epidural or don't, or if your baby is pushed or lifted. Yoga's gift is that you truly recognize the profound power in your body.

Yoga's gift is that you truly recognize the profound power in your body.

labor and birth

WISDOM
the stages and phases of vaginal birth

With pregnancy, the size of your uterus changes. It grows from the size of a pear to a watermelon. At the end of pregnancy, the top of your uterus (called the fundus) extends to your rib cage. And yes, your other organs shift to make room for your growing baby and uterus.

As birth looms, there are some signs that labor is approaching: You might feel pelvic pressure or as if you have more room in the upper part of your torso. You may have increased vaginal discharge or a "bloody show" (which is the bloody mucus of the cervical plug that loosens or comes out). You may experience a sudden burst of energy (a desire to clean and nest). You could deal with gastrointestinal distress or diarrhea the days or hours before labor begins. Most likely, your water (the amniotic sac) will break after labor has started. For about 15 percent of birth parents, water breaks before the onset of contractions. (Alexandra is in that latter group: her water broke in the bathroom of her favorite coffee shop when no other signs of labor had begun!)

You may experience a sudden burst of energy (a desire to clean and nest).

One important star of the labor show is your cervix. Viewed from the vaginal canal, your cervix looks like a doughnut. Your cervix has an important job in the weeks, days, or hours before labor begins; it must soften (ripen), thin (efface), and open (dilate). During or prior to the onset of labor, you can ask your doctor or midwife to share how dilated you are, or—if knowing this feels like it would add to your concerns of stress—you might ask for that information to be withheld.

Medically, labor gets broken into three stages. The first stage is the onset of labor until cervical dilation is complete. The second stage of labor is complete dilation until the delivery of your baby. This is often called the "pushing" stage, and this stage of labor might last minutes or hours! The third stage of labor is the delivery of your placenta. Once your baby is born, the placenta will arrive five to thirty minutes later. Abdominal massage (to encourage your uterus to contract and prevent postpartum hemorrhage) by a midwife or nurse may occur afterward.

That first stage, though, is where most of the "labor" of laboring takes place. It's the stage you're likely to be in the longest. Within the first stage of labor, there are three distinct phases. Early or latent labor begins with the onset of labor and continues until your cervix is dilated up to five to six centimeters. Regardless of your ultimate birth setting, you will likely labor at home for much of this first phase. During this time, your care provider will likely encourage you to rest, if possible, eat and drink, relax, and shower or bathe.

Active labor begins around 5 to 6 centimeters of cervical dilation and continues until 7 to 8 centimeters. If you're moving to a different setting (like a hospital or birth center), you might be told to follow the four-one-one rule: that means your contractions are coming regularly four minutes apart, each one lasting at least one minute, and this has been ongoing for about one hour. (Care practitioners might differ on this and say five-one-one rule, or even three-one-one rule.) During active labor, you will likely want to use massage, a yoga ball, a transcutaneous electrical nerve stimulation (TENS) unit, nitrous oxide, an epidural, or other measures for the management of discomfort.

The transition phase comes next, and it may be the most intense phase of your labor. You may say things like "I can't do this anymore." This is the phase where doulas and partners may need to be especially reassuring and grounding, so you may want to talk through how to handle this phase in advance.

There's no rule for how long these phases last. People who have delivered a baby before often move more quickly through dilation and labor. Some birthing people progress more quickly than others. Some birthing people "stall" at a certain stage, and then dilate very quickly. Not all labor looks the same. Common variations of labor include prodromal labor (labor that starts and stops before fully active labor begins), a prolonged active phase, contractions that do not become regular, and a prolonged second stage (prolonged pushing).

Between dilating to 10 centimeters and feeling an urge to push, some women and birth parents experience a "rest and be thankful stage," where they are fully dilated but do not feel an urge to push. Instead, they feel relaxed and may even fall asleep. According to the book *Our Bodies, Ourselves: Pregnancy and Birth*, "Research suggests that the length of time before the baby is born is the same if you allow one hour of 'passive descent' of the baby (when you relax and don't consciously try to push) or you start pushing immediately after you are fully dilated."

All vaginal births are unique and may follow a circuitous route. First-time mothers and birthing parents can labor for hours or days—and both of those are normal. As you move toward birth, it's helpful to understand not just the phases and stages of birth, but that your particular birth experience may vary greatly.

RELATE
Alexandra on her birth preferences, birth story, and birth meaning

I have always been hospital phobic. I don't like needles, and I have broken into tears more than once at having my blood drawn. Or, more fun, I grow faint and weak, feeling extraordinarily vulnerable. On my visits to the doctor during my pregnancy with my daughter, I admit I often felt more anxious about the requisite blood draw than I did about my growing baby's health: That's how illogical these fears are. Obviously, thinking about birthing, I had some strong preferences!

I was fearful of a hospital birth (and the needles it may involve), and I made plans to deliver my daughter in a birthing center. At the birthing center, continuous fetal monitoring was not required. Being hooked up to an IV was not required. Eating and drinking were allowed and encouraged. I could walk around, go outside, even take laps in the parking lot (all of which I inevitably did). Epidurals weren't possible, although morphine, nitrous oxide, and nonmedical pain relief like TENS units and hydrotherapy were available. The birth center rooms looked like cozy bedrooms; the medical equipment was confined to a quiet corner. In the room I ended up birthing in, the walls were a soothing blue, and there was a sweet picture of a cheery mermaid hung next to the door.

When I shared my birth plans with a trusted friend (who also happened to be pregnant), she was horrified that I would choose to birth my child in what she deemed a perilous environment, without the medical capabilities she felt were necessary for a safe delivery. I remember being surprised: Labor and delivery felt like innately, intuitively safe experiences to me, and I didn't feel worried about my safety or my baby's safety. Somehow, that hadn't really crossed my mind. I just knew I didn't want the stress and anxiety of having a needle in my arm as I brought my child into the world. Needles disconnect me from myself, and I wanted to stay present and connected during what was surely one of the most important days of my life. I didn't want to hear machines beeping. I didn't want to be confined to a bed.

My daughter's birth was idyllic in many ways. It was a long birth—I call it my birthing weekend—but I had the birth that I think I must have needed. Through hours of stalled contractions and then sped-up birth (thanks to herbs, and—much less pleasant—thanks to castor oil), it was mostly me and my partner. Birth centers aren't teeming with people. And although nurses and midwives came in to check on us and my parents were ready and nearby, it was my partner who cared for me, supported me, encouraged me, and made me feel deeply loved and held. He showed up for me hour after hour, late through the night and early in the morning—always there when I most needed him. He was completely present with me at my most base and most vulnerable—he didn't shy away from any part of it. He stayed by my side through the growing waves of early labor and then in the stranger, hazy parts of labor when I was reduced to my most primal self: walking, squatting, moaning, but no longer using words. In between contractions in active labor, he would guide me to an enormous pile of pillows he'd lumped onto the birthing bed and massage my feet and calves and legs. In my memory, this went on for hours. Me, walking, squatting, moaning. Him, guiding me, massaging me, helping me back up to weather another contraction (which felt best when I was on my feet and moving). Through one of the most challenging experiences of my life, he was there with me for every moment.

I often consider that maybe there was something about my daughter's birth that my spiritual self needed. If you'd asked me before I gave birth if I felt my partner loved me, I would have offered a resounding yes. But to see and feel and experience his presence in the fire with me cemented his love; it showed me his love in action. It felt like proof that he would be there, no matter the hardship or hurdle. In order to move into confident motherhood with my partner by my side, maybe there was an intuitive part of me that needed us to find ourselves as a team during our child's birth.

labor and birth

But also, that's how I make sense of the birth experience I had: It's how I create my meaning for it, as we all create our own meanings for the profound birth experiences we have. That's the neat thing about birth stories: We get to weave them into the threads of the existing theories and mythologies we have about our lives and selves. Whatever birth experiences we have become fodder for the themes of our personal stories as we make sense of the events that unfolded when our children arrived into the world.

About my birth, though, mostly, I'm just glad I didn't have to be in a medicalized environment. My daughter arrived safely—not in a hospital—and happily, there were no needles involved in her birth.

WISDOM
make some noise

According to Ina May Gaskin, the pioneer of the modern midwifery movement in America, muscles that have a purpose of holding something in (like the cervix, bladder, and rectum) are waiting for a prompt to let go and allow whatever they are holding to come out. Pressure is often the prompt that encourages these muscles to relax and dispel their contents.

These sphincter muscles are mostly involuntary and they have specific characteristics: particularly, that they all work best in comfortable and private environments. For this reason, feeling safe, cared for, and supported is important for a vaginal birth. It's helpful to consider in advance of your birth how much your environment can be controlled: Will you be able to have low lighting, essential oils, music, drinks, or whatever else makes you feel most secure?

Gaskin also notes that the muscles of the mouth and jaw directly correlate to the muscles of the sphincter: If one area is relaxed, so is the other. As we've noted previously regarding the pelvic floor (in Chapter 4), a released, softened pelvic floor is important during childbirth. One way to loosen your jaw, face, and mouth is to make some noise. And if your jaw is relaxed, then ostensibly, so is your pelvic floor.

The most common noise of childbirth is moaning. If you can moan in a deep, guttural, low tone, you're expelling your breath effectively, which is another key for childbirth. Noisemaking, breathing out, pelvic floor relaxation: These things all work in tandem. If you are moaning low and deep, you're helping your baby make the slow transition down and out, and you're channeling the energy and sensations that are coming up as a result.

Loud breathing is another type of common noise in labor and birth. Your yoga breathwork has prepared you to think about breathing, but once you're in active labor the most important thing is not *how* you breathe, but that you *continue* to breathe (rather than holding your breath). It's okay to sigh out, pant, moan, or breathe noisily in any way that feels good. According to Carleen McKenna, Certified Nurse Midwife, many people tense their entire body during a contraction. Focusing on exhaling and relaxing your shoulders, face, and eyes as a contraction is ending is a practice she often initiates with her patients. "People hold incredible amounts of tension/stress/fear/anxiety/trauma in the pelvic floor, similar to what we are all aware we hold in our shoulders and neck," she says. "There is so much benefit from breath work with pelvic floor relaxation."

You might cry during your labor: That's not an uncommon reaction to a lack of sleep or an onslaught of sensations. As you probably know from experience, we often cry when we feel emotional release. This sometimes happens in yoga! Crying is another type of noise you may make in labor, and it's a good one: it means you are letting out emotions, feelings, sensations, fears.

Singing, chanting, or repeating phrases is common, and at some point, if you are using a mantra or mantras, they may disintegrate into mumbling or murmuring as labor intensifies. You might hold onto the threads of these intentional phrases, but the phrases themselves might fade away from actual language.

When you arrive at the pushing stage, your moans may get even lower, and you might make grunting, groaning noises. These noises are productive: Consider that if you were lifting a big weight in a gym or otherwise doing something that required a lot of exertion, you would likely groan or grunt. It's the same thing here.

Whatever your noises are, you are going to make noise as you labor and deliver. One way to get comfortable with noisemaking in labor is to make some noise *before* labor begins.

labor and birth

REFLECT
A, E, I, O, U: the value of vowel sounds and vocal toning

We love to chant Sanskrit and English, but this chanting exercise is even more basic; it's the chanting of vowel sounds. This may be a useful practice in early labor that you can harken back to as labor gets more intense. Or you might practice while still pregnant, to discover a comfortable vowel sound that you can use during your birth.

Start by softening your throat—you might swallow once or twice. Keep this sensation of an open throat tone for the entire length of your exhale, always following a deep inhalation. (If you are practicing vocal toning and vowel chanting in active labor, it may feel more challenging to take one deep inhalation, in which case, take a few smaller inhalations before you exhale out and chant.)

This practice is a vowel sound exercise. After each inhalation, you chant out a vowel sound.

Inhale, and then chant out A, as in the word *play*.

Inhale, and then chant out E, as in the word *me*.

Inhale, and chant out I, as in *find*.

Inhale and chant out O, as in *oh* or *om*.

Inhale and chant out U, as in *uh* or *bug*.

If you explore this before labor or during early labor, you might notice a preferred sound that you can use again as labor intensifies. Go with your intuitive sound: There is no wrong or right sound to chant. What allows you to relax your body, breathe out, and find pleasant focus?

WISDOM
the power of birth support

Laura Lundegard, perinatal yoga teacher and doula, describes the role of her doula work.

As a doula, I provide prenatal visits, support through labor, and postpartum appointments. Each client I work with gets a guidebook that walks them through a very basic overview of childbirth and newborn-care education filled with my own tips, tricks, and recommendations.

My prenatal support includes an initial home visit where I sit down with the family and review their preferences for birth. We discuss their dreams, hopes, fears, and concerns. In this first appointment, my goal is to really get to know the mother or birth parent and know exactly what she wants for her labor and delivery. Or, if she is uncertain, I will give her the information she needs, including benefits, risks, and alternatives to help her make an informed decision. Those decisions can be tabled so she can research on her own more or discuss them with her care provider.

In that same discussion we also review the unexpected. As a doula, I want to be sure that the mom, birth partner (if applicable), and myself are all on the same page in terms of birth preferences. The remainder of the first appointment is spent discussing comfort measures that we can try during labor, going over possible laboring positions, and discussing how to cope with sensation and with surges. (I don't like using the word *pain*. I prefer *sensation,* which can help rewire the brain and our preconceived notions around labor being "painful" or scary. Similarly, I don't like using the word *contraction,* I prefer *surge,* as it suggests power!)

After that appointment, I send the mom or birth parent all the notes I've taken about her preferences. From there, she creates her birth preferences (or plan). In the following prenatal appointment, I address any questions or fears about labor, birth, or newborn care left over from the first appointment, and then we review postpartum and newborn education.

The final prenatal visit focuses either entirely on comfort measures for labor, or it can be a visit with the mom-to-be to a prenatal care appointment with her OB or midwife, so that way I have the ability to meet some of the team prior to her labor.

During labor, I ask the mother or birth parent to call me one or two hours before she thinks she will need me, even if it's the middle of the night! When I initially receive the call, I check in to see how she is feeling, and I will typically get details about her surges, if her water has broken, and if she has called her other providers. From that information I'll assess for myself where she likely is in her labor and then let her know my estimated time of arrival. In the typical case (a low-risk, healthy pregnancy with a planned unmedicated hospital delivery), I'll labor with the mother at home as long as we can before going to the hospital. While at her home, we will utilize various

labor and birth

comfort measures, from massage, birth balls, TENS units, cool towels, heating pads, music, breath work, meditation, and mantra to help her cope. As a birth worker, the comfort measure component is highly instinctual and intuitive for me: the moment I walk into the home, I quickly assess where the mother is holding tension, assess how she is currently coping with her surges, and I work to help her drop into her body and let herself surrender.

While laboring with the mother, I will time surges until they reach the four-one-one pattern. In the case of a hospital delivery, I'll instruct the partner to pack the car and call the provider, and then I'll help mom into the car during a break between surges. Upon arrival at the hospital, I continue to labor with the mother and also advocate for her birth plan when or if it's challenged by hospital staff or labor and delivery nurses. I keep supporting the mother through her delivery and remain her advocate even after the baby has been born. Once the baby has arrived, I help with breastfeeding and getting the first latch, and stay until everyone is settled in the postpartum recovery room. Once everything is taken care of, I head off to rest, and then check in with them when I wake up the next day.

MOVE
partner support yoga for labor

Partner support in yoga might look like hand holding and squeezing, leg support and bracing, low-back massage, or foot rubs. The yoga asana of labor may look like others moving their bodies to support yours. Following are some movement ideas that many have found helpful during labor. A birth ball (and a partner or doula to participate in the shared exercise) are props required here.

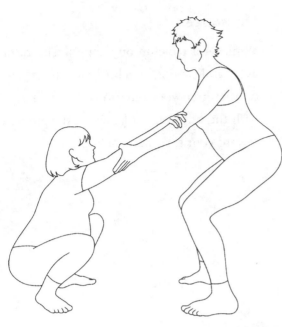

Supported squat

Grab the forearms of your birth support person and have them grab hold of yours. Settle into a squatting position, using their counterweight to help balance and stabilize you, allowing you to sink more deeply into the squatting position.

Shaking the apples

Come into a tabletop position or a supported puppy pose. Have your support person gently grab the back of your thighs with their whole hand and jiggle them back and forth. This is a good move to practice while you're still pregnant. It can feel silly and a bit weird but can be a really helpful tool while in active labor.

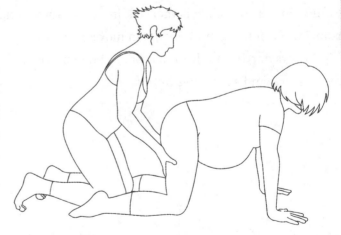

labor and birth

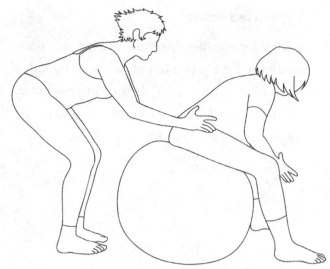

Hip squeeze

While in a tabletop or puppy position, or even while sitting on a birth ball, have your partner grab your outermost hip area and, with the full weight of their body, press in toward your sacrum from both sides.

Yoga ball rolling

Sitting on a birth ball, whether holding on to something or someone or nothing, find rhythm in movement, circling your hips or swaying from side to side, or any other movement that feels natural and supportive to you.

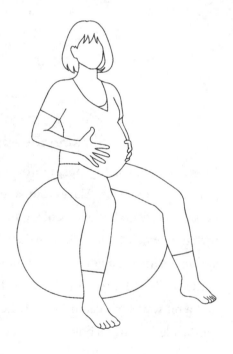

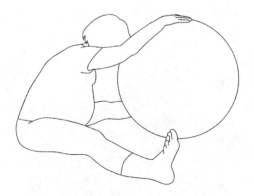

Yoga ball seated head support

Sitting on the floor, position your legs wide, and lean forward, wrapping your arms around the yoga ball. Lean your head against it, if possible. If the ball feels like it's going to roll away from you or feels unstable in any way, prop it against a wall first.

Partner sways

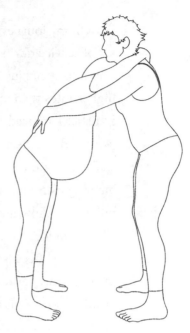

In a standing position, wrap your arms around your partner or support person's neck and lean into them, giving as much of your body weight to them as you can. Sway from side to side, middle-school dance style.

REFLECT
birth mantra as ritual during labor

In her writing on birth, renowned physical therapist and doula Penny Simkin talks a lot about the three Rs: relaxation, rhythm, and ritual. Mantra is another powerful tool for both rhythm and personally significant ritual. In yoga, we often chant repeated phrases (like *om*) at the start or end of a practice. This ritual in yoga serves to set the tone for the practice and can sometimes serve as an intention. In this same way, mantra in labor can serve as an intention.

Here are some positive mantras for labor:

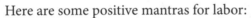

My body was made for this.
Each contraction brings my baby closer.
I am drawing on the energy of those before me.
My baby and I are working together.
I trust my body.
I am strong.
This is what's happening now.
Open, down, out.

WISDOM
doula work as social justice

Quanisha Callwood, birth and postpartum doula and mom of two little ones, shares a bit about her experience supporting Black and Brown birth parents and mothers in labor and birth.

labor and birth

On my journey to becoming a doula, I soon realized that it was more than just an act of service during such a vulnerable time in the lives of women. It was also a transition into social justice work. Black and Brown women continue to die at significantly higher rates than white women. My work as a doula connected me directly with that statistic. I noticed the positive impact of having a birth doula present at births and would often reflect on the care provided because of it. During births I remind hospital staff that I am a support to them as well. I emphasize the importance of utilizing the birthing plan that my client and I have created. I approach matters from a warm standpoint and allow hospital staff to ask any questions that they may have regarding my client's choices. Often, my clients feel empowered and eager to stand up for their rights and wishes. Because of this approach and the education provided to my client, birthing outcomes for my clients and their babies have been positive. We have experienced beautiful moments and when moments aren't as positive, we can reflect on them and safely refuse unwarranted services from an evidence-based approach.

BREATHE
breathe to relax your pelvic floor

Both of the following breath practices incorporate mouth movements and noises that release tension in the face, jaw, and mouth during the exhalation. Using these breath practices in early and active labor can be a helpful way to continue to relax your face, body, and pelvic floor.

horse lips' breath

Start with the concept of relaxation. Relax your face and jaw as much as you can and take a few breaths in through your nose and out through your mouth. Then, allow your lips to come together softly and breathe in through your nose. As you breathe out, relax your mouth, and "flutter" your lips, making a sound familiar from horses, called a "nicker." Take three-to-five breaths in this manner and check in with the muscles of your pelvic floor as you explore this breath.

lion's breath

Lion's breath is a classic pranayama practice, and it is often used in the fiery moments of a yoga practice. Here, you can use it during the fiery moments of your labor. To practice this breath, take a deep breath in through your nose. To exhale, open your mouth, and stick out your tongue, turning your gaze toward the ceiling. Allow the muscles of your face to stretch as you widen your mouth. On the breath out, make a sound like "ha!" extending the "aa" part of that word.

RELATE

Kate, mom to two boys, shares a breath practice that was particularly helpful to her during labor.

The most vivid memory of using breathwork I learned in prenatal yoga outside of the studio is during labor with my second child. In prenatal yoga, we practiced specific breaths including lion's breath. It made me roll my eyes a bit during class as it felt silly, and I'd already given birth before! I had *this* and didn't need *that*. Enter my second labor which was so different than my first. Needing Pitocin and having strong, fast contractions made lion's breath my best friend. My partner and that silly breath got me through hours of labor to meet my little guy.

MOVE
move to serve your labor

If you are able to move around during labor, you may try pacing, squatting, or rocking on a yoga ball through contractions. Giving birth in a birth center allowed Alexandra ample opportunity to find her own birth rhythm: She favored squatting while holding on to a counter for additional support, or pacing the room. The day after her daughter was born, the sorest parts of her body were her quads, feet, and calves!

But being confined to a bed or table doesn't mean you can't explore the value of rhythm and ritual. With an IV pole attached to her wrist, heart rate monitors strapped

labor and birth

to her belly, Lauren found rhythm and ritual through moving in time to some of her favorite kirtan music. You might drop your knees side to side, squeeze and release your hands into fists, scrunch up and soften your face, or shrug and release your shoulders in response to discomfort, anxiety, or new and strange sensations. Your rhythm can be your trusted breath; you've been connecting to it through your entire pregnancy! Wherever you are, whatever is happening, if you are alert and awake, you can find your breath—that breath can offer you tempo, pattern, and flow, even when your body is numb, still, or in surgery.

partner support yoga for labor

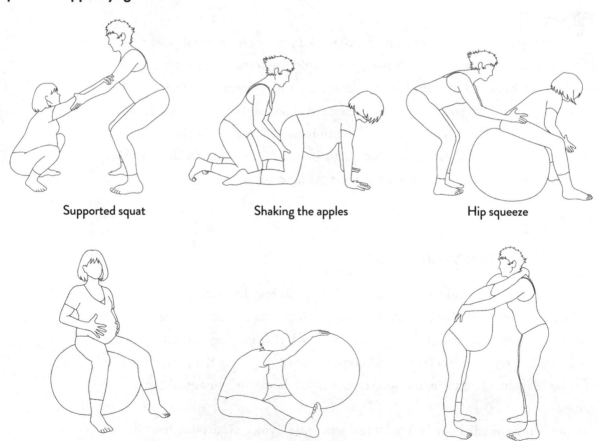

Supported squat   Shaking the apples   Hip squeeze

Yoga ball rolling   Yoga ball seated head support   Partner sways

when things go exactly as planned (and when they don't)

Birth plans are tricky. They're good to have, and they're good to let go. Meg Berreth, Certified Nurse Midwife, says, "Preparing for birth is like preparing for an ocean voyage. You can stock the ship, build a strong vessel, and have powerful sails and a great crew . . . But you can't control the weather, or the sea." Just as change is the only constant in life, confronting the unexpected is perhaps the only guarantee in childbirth. Depending on how far you had to veer off course, you might be feeling any number of things about your birth experience. It will take time to emotionally integrate and process your labor and birth.

We are not assuming that you're reading this chapter because you had a cesarean birth, although some of the information and experiences we offer here will be devoted to that type of birth. Many cesarean births are planned, and even if you had one that was unplanned, your experience may have been positive. On the flip side, if you had a vaginal birth, it may or may not feel like things went "as planned." The use of forceps, vaginal tearing, or moments of fetal or maternal distress may have all left their mark. There may be residual trauma associated with your child's birth, regardless of the details, process, or how it took place. There is an assumption that vaginal births are always happy births and cesarean births are always negative. From our own births and our discussions with other birthing people in the context of birth processing and yoga workshops, we know this isn't true. What is true is that if you felt out of control in your birth narrative, if you felt like things happened suddenly and without clear explanation, or if you felt frightened for your safety or your child's safety, then you have likely arrived on this side of the birth experience with a lot to process, make peace with, and work through.

What is true is that if you felt out of control ..., then you have likely arrived on this side of the birth experience with a lot to process, make peace with, and work through.

Even if you feel like things went smoothly in your child's birth, birth is an evolved, often lengthy, and nuanced life event that has attendant emotional moments. Everyone who has been through birth needs to process it, and a trusted care provider or therapist can help. Peer support and connection (the kind that you might find in a birth processing workshop or postpartum yoga class) can also be a valuable way to understand or reconceive your birth experience in the context of others' experiences.

It might also be useful to think of your birth experience in a general way rather than focus on details: Details of things which "went wrong" can feel haunting; self-blame is unhelpful and detrimental. If your child's birth did not go as you hoped, take the time to sit with that grief. You may also feel a lot of paradoxical emotions: relief that you and your baby are fine, fear of birthing again, sadness that you didn't experience the birth you wanted, profound joy, and profound loss.

One especially challenging aspect of birth experiences is that whether you have a "good one" or a "bad one" might be a factor of luck, or it may be connected to the area of the country you live in, the quality of the hospital you birthed in (lower-income birth parents are more likely to receive medical interventions), or your race. There are discrepancies in treatment for birthing people, and often those discrepancies are rooted in systemic racism or economic inequity. In short, there are many factors to consider when you analyze how your birth experience unfolded.

REFLECT
inhale, heal

Processing your birth experience is going to take a while, whether birth went exactly as you planned it or whether it took a very circuitous route. It's important to remember that you have also just been born into motherhood or parenthood, and that however your child's life began is but one small moment in a very long relationship that you will have with your child. It's hard to conceive of time passing and the freshness of emotions in this experience fading or being threaded into your larger life story, but that will happen. For now, it's enough to have faith that you are okay now, regardless of what happened, and you will be okay later, too. Sit quietly in a comfortable chair (with or without your baby in your arms). Take full, deep breaths. On the inhale, imagine you are breathing in healing energy: healing energy for your body, your heart, your spirit. On the exhale, imagine you are breathing out heaviness: heaviness of emotion, the heaviness of repair, the heaviness of effort and work.

RELATE
the innate wisdom of your baby

In many books about birth and particularly books about birth and yoga, there is little mention of the possibility of a cesarean delivery. In our Western culture, and particularly in our yogic culture within that Western culture, vaginal and, particularly, vaginal births without medical intervention, are glorified. So many of the exercises, breathing practices, and meditations envision a vaginal delivery, yet 32 percent of births in the United States are cesarean.

During one particularly poignant moment in the very first yoga teacher training that we led, one of our guests, a renowned, mystical massage therapist was touting the benefits of prenatal massage for optimal fetal positioning, the benefits of vaginal delivery for mom and baby, and the natural oxytocin that is produced during an unmedicated birth.

labor and birth

One of the students asked a question and preceded the question by acknowledging her own recent cesarean birth, in an almost apologetic way. Without missing a beat, our presenter answered her question but not before saying, "Isn't it incredible that babies just *know* how birth will work best for them? He knew he needed to be lifted out. That's wonderful." We both still get chills thinking about the powerful affirmation this kind and wise woman delivered. It wasn't toxic positivity or the platitude of "Well, you're both safe now." It was a recognition that babies have innate wisdom, too. The student who asked the question radiated relief, and we know that that moment went far in helping her process her own feelings about her birth experience.

Babies may know best. Cesarean birth can be the very best way for your baby to make their earthside debut. And birth can be powerful and empowering, no matter what path it takes.

RELATE
Lauren's birth story

One of the reasons that women attend prenatal yoga classes is in the hope that the poses, breathwork, and meditation will equip them with the tools for a successful birth experience. That idea of having a "successful birth experience" can be really weighted, loaded down with input from friends and relatives, societal pressures, internal hopes and fears, and the experiences, both positive and negative, true, and less so, that an individual has encountered over the course of their pregnancy. *Every* type of birth is criticized. If there is an ideal birth, as envisioned by a subset of our privileged Western culture, it includes little intervention, pain (if that's even what it's called) managed/ embraced by nonmedicinal means, a nonclinical setting, a vaginal delivery, immediate skin-to-skin contact, and a profound love and affinity for breastfeeding. *Whew!* That is one tall order.

As a prenatal yoga instructor, I have battled the imposter complex when it comes to my own birth experience. I didn't give birth to either of my children in a candlelit water bath at home, emitting only the sound of *om* as their heads crowned, basking in the rosy glow of oxytocin as they were placed in my arms. Instead, surrounded by at least a dozen medical professionals in a cold, fluorescent-lit operating room, my first feeling when I saw my son was not one of pure bliss but, rather, extreme nausea. I was amazed to see him but mostly overwhelmed by the strong desire to not throw up on my newborn's head. I didn't get skin-to-skin contact, as more attention was being focused on my uterus, which was, as my midwife had informed me before the operation, "kaput." As sometimes happens during cesarean operations, when a person has been on Pitocin for a long time, my uterus was so worn out that it wouldn't contract back without external intervention. A team of residents streamed into the operating room for a glimpse of the attending surgeon removing my uterus from my body and tying it up, Thanksgiving-turkey style, so that my uterus would cease expelling its contents and realize that its job was finally done.

Nauseous first glimpse aside, I didn't see Simon until several hours after he was born. After his delivery, I basked, instead, in the glow of morphine, the bliss of a catheter (for a bladder that had seen constant action for nine months), and the delight of Gatorade. In the wee hours of the morning when the nurse asked if I needed anything, it dawned on me that I hadn't actually held my son. I had lost 3 liters of blood, been in surgery for hours, given my family quite a scare, and still had no feeling in my lower body. My physiological state was far from ideal. Holding Simon, however, was perfect.

I didn't struggle with my own birth experience until someone told me that I should. A visitor hugged me and, with tears in her eyes, told me how sorry she was that I "had to have all of those interventions." With just a few words, a small seed of doubt took hold. Did I do everything I could? Was I just not strong enough? Did my body not understand its role? I hadn't been sorry. Until I was.

Questions have risen, intermittently, in the years since Simon was born. By talking to other women, writing, yoga, and (mostly) experiencing motherhood (and how much of it doesn't go "as planned"), I've been able to release a great deal of the

labor and birth

"should" as far as my own role in my son's birth. It took some time to get here—to a place of peace, with a sense of authenticity that, even though I gave birth in a way that I never anticipated, my experience is every bit as valid.

WISDOM
what to know about cesarean birth

Cesarean births can be planned in advance, and they can also happen after labor has begun. Depending on whether you have already received anesthesia in the form of an epidural or another method of delivery, you may or may not be able to walk into the operating room. You are generally allowed to have one support person in the room with you, though that will depend on the protocol followed by your hospital.

At the start of surgery, an incision is made, usually in a four-to six-inch horizontal line at or around the pubic hair line. An additional four-to six-inch uterine incision will be made in order to gain access to the baby and the placenta. After the second incision is made, suction will be used to draw out amniotic fluid. Depending on the position of the baby, your baby's head will be delivered first, then shoulders and the rest of the baby. (In the case of a breech delivery—a common reason for cesarean births—your baby's bottom, torso, and legs will be out first.) Because fluid accumulates in the baby's lungs and is not forced out as it usually is during vaginal birth, the operating physician will suction your baby's mouth to remove any remaining fluid so that normal breathing can begin.

Thinking about the *possibility* of a cesarean birth while envisioning your birth experience prior to birth can be helpful. Talking with others who have had their own babies this way can be useful in determining how you might need help and support after birth.

If you've delivered via cesarean birth, you have also had major abdominal surgery. It is incredible that people can have their babies this way and also be expected to care for them! Can you imagine if someone had their appendix removed (a much smaller incision, by the way) and then someone handed them a puppy? *Insane.* Our culture and society don't set us up very well for this. Creating a support network that works for you and your family is so important. It might be helpful to make a list of different aspects of life that might be challenging with a new baby and ill-advised after abdominal surgery.

WISDOM
cesarean care through scar massage

When cesarean surgery occurs, both internal and external scar tissue forms as a result of the two incisions made. When surgery occurs, the fascia is also cut. Fascia is the thin casing of connective tissue that surrounds and holds every muscle, organ, blood vessel, bone, and nerve fiber in place. It usually runs in an ordered, horizontal way, allowing underlying tissues to glide and move easily. After fascia has been cut, when it reforms, it grows in a more haphazard way and can more easily bind (i.e., adhere) to what underlies it—usually muscle or organ tissue. When these *adhesions* form, they can cause less mobility and possibly more pain. Massaging the scar tissue surrounding your cesarean scar as well as the healed scar itself can be helpful and effective. Wait until your scar has completely healed before beginning these massage exercises. If your scar is still in the process of healing, you can help stimulate sensation by lightly brushing a clean cotton ball over the area.

When your scar has completely healed (usually by four to six weeks postpartum), you can begin massaging the area to encourage increased blood flow and decrease adhesions. This massage can even be helpful and effective many *years* after scar tissue has formed. Lauren just recently purchased more castor oil for massage, and her "baby" is seven years old. Castor oil is an appropriate oil to use, as are coconut, almond oil, and other neutral oils.

- Place your index and middle fingers two to three inches away from the scar and stretch skin up and down around the entire scar. Move side to side, up and down, and then clockwise and counterclockwise.
- Place two to three fingers directly on the scar, starting at the center, and press the scar one inch in one direction (up or down) and hold for ten to fifteen seconds. Repeat this, moving out to one end of the scar and then, again from the center, moving out to the other end of the scar. You can play around with moving in up-and-down and circular motions, but hold the stretch for several breaths, regardless of the direction you choose.
- Finally, pinching your scar tissue between your index finger and thumb, lift the tissue away from your body and roll the scar between your fingers for ten to fifteen seconds. Move along the length of the scar, repeating this as you go.

labor and birth

MOVE
yoga after cesarean birth

If you delivered your baby through cesarean birth, this is an excellent yoga practice to help you explore the sensations of your healing abdomen, gently engage the core muscles, and observe how your changed body feels.

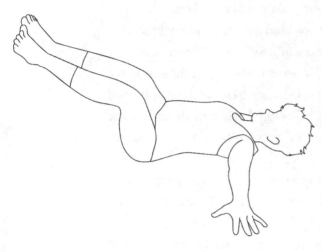

Knees in line—one side and then the other

Lie on your back and bend your knees and then lift your feet off the floor. With your shins parallel to the ground and your thighs perpendicular, draw your navel toward your spine, to whatever extent you can, and, keeping your knees in line, slowly lower them a few inches to the right. Reengage your core by drawing your navel back to your spine again and then bring your legs back up and slowly to the other side. Repeat this three to five times on either side.

Tabletop bird dog

Come up to a tabletop position. From here, stretch your right leg back, keeping your foot on the ground and drawing your navel to your spine. Slowly begin to lift your right leg up. This could be one or two inches, or all the way up to the

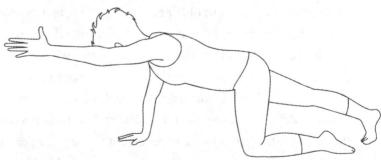

height of your hip if you're able to maintain length in your lower back and engagement of your low belly muscles. Take it slow. To play with balance and further core engagement, you could also extend your left arm alongside your left ear. Breathe here for a few rounds of breath before switching sides.

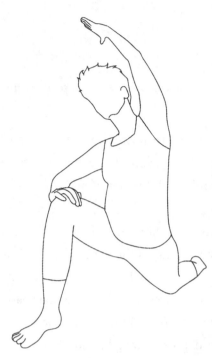

Low lunge

From a tabletop position, walk your hands over to the left slightly and then draw your right foot forward and place it to the outside of your hands. Place both hands on the top of your right thigh. Press your hands into your right leg and forward as you lift up through your sternum. Practice sinking your right hip and left thigh toward the floor to explore a stretch of your incision. You might feel a slight pulling or tugging sensation, and if there's any pain, you can use your back knee as a kind of brake, energetically drawing it forward toward your front foot. After you've explored some subtle movement forward and back a few times, switch sides slowly.

Knees-down plank

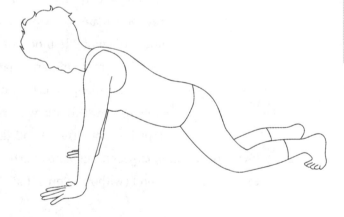

Come back into a tabletop position. Walk your knees back a few inches and keep your shoulders over your wrists, drawing your navel toward your spine as you do so. Lengthen your tailbone toward your heels. You might play around with bending your elbows slightly and lowering your chest toward the floor a few inches and then back up. Or you might just hold this variation on a plank pose, keeping your lower belly muscles active and engaged. Rest when you need to and slowly build up strength in this position.

labor and birth

WISDOM
motherhood: hard in all circumstances

Felice Reddy, PhD, perinatal therapist, shares her reflections on working with people after they've arrived at motherhood.

The thing I hear most often while doing therapy with postpartum women and moms with older kids is something along the lines of "Everyone else is better at this/struggling less/liking it more than me." We need to debunk the myths and normalize the struggle!

If I could write reminder cue cards for all moms, these are some of the sentiments I would communicate: Motherhood that includes balancing all the demands, expectations, worries, and appearances is difficult largely because of societal norms and harmful constructs. There is an expectation that women will love their baby immediately—this is not always *true*. We are told that strong marriages can weather parenting; in fact, the degree of tangible and emotional help and support by the nonbirthing parent greatly predicts marital distress and maternal depression. Many women think that if they don't have a diagnosable mood or anxiety condition they are "fine"; in fact, there is a spectrum, and many women are suffering without knowing they can get help. Society would have us believe that surviving is good enough—most moms will sacrifice their own hobbies, goals, relationships for motherhood and think that is what is required. In fact, if we lowered pressure, expectations, and martyrdom, many women would find a way to thrive in motherhood (without "doing it all").

There is an expectation that women will love their baby immediately—this is not always true.

yoga after cesarean birth

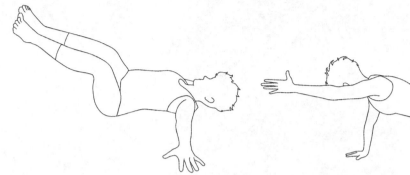

Knees in line—one side and then the other

Tabletop bird dog

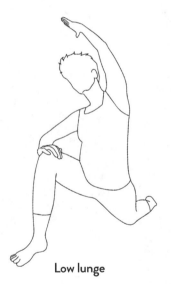

Low lunge

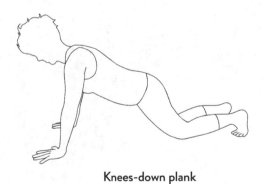

Knees-down plank

Part Four

postpartum

Chapter Eight
your yoga now

Congratulations! You have a baby, and you are no longer pregnant. How are you feeling? The early days of being a mom or birth parent can be filled with lots of challenges: lack of sleep, disconnection from your body, exhaustion, hormone shifts, and change, change, change. If you're crying a lot, that's normal. If you're laughing a lot, that's normal. If you feel flooded with love and oxytocin, that's normal. If you feel frustrated and scared, that's normal.

The medical community defines the postpartum period by identifying three distinct phases:

The *acute postpartum period* is the first six to twelve hours after your baby has been born. This is a time of a lot of big changes, and because there are still some potential maternal health concerns during this time, you will likely be monitored by a care provider, midwife, nurse, or doctor.

The second phase is the *subacute postpartum period*, which can last between two to six weeks after you give birth. Your body is undergoing really big changes in terms of blood flow, metabolism, hormones and emotions, and pelvic floor recovery.

The final postpartum phase that the medical community identifies is the *delayed postpartum period*, which can last up to six months. In literature on being postpartum, though, it is commonly acknowledged that some healing takes place well beyond the six-month mark, and some changes of birth are permanent.

postpartum

We think that the word *postpartum* is a label you can use for as long as it feels applicable, medical definition aside. Many of us nurse well beyond six months, don't have regular periods for up to a year, and we certainly don't feel "back to our normal selves" even two to three years after we became mothers and parents.

Let's unpack that idea, anyway. The point of the poses and breath practices in these chapters is not to transport you and your body back to who or what you were before you became a mom. Your prebaby body may be eventually accessible to you, or your body may forever look and feel different. When you went from prepubescent through puberty, your body changed, your personality changed, your needs changed. So, too, as you move from your maiden self to motherhood, you've gone through a shift, a change, a reevaluation of what matters. The reproductive psychiatrist Alexandra Sacks, MD, has written extensively about the concept of *matrescence*. Matrescence is the major life transition that occurs when a mother goes through pregnancy and gives birth. In a *New York Times* article called "Birth of a Mother," Sacks points out that "becoming a mother is an identity shift, and one of the most significant physical and psychological changes a woman will ever experience."

Your prebaby body may be eventually accessible to you, or your body may forever look and feel different.

All people who become parents go through a tremendous shift, but Sacks reminds us that birthing people and "women who go through the hormonal changes of pregnancy" are the ones who "have a specific neurobiological experience." In short, the changes you've gone through physically, mentally, spiritually, and hormonally can't be reversed. And they certainly can't be reduced to "get your body back."

We want to be clear, though, that we know you want to feel comfortable in your body, and in the days, weeks, and months after you become a mom or parent, you may feel like your body is a strange being that happens to be carting around your (exhausted) spirit. You may be carrying more weight now than before you were pregnant. It can take up to eight weeks for your uterus to reduce back to its prepregnancy size.

In our culture, we often focus on the baby, not the transition that the mother or birth parent just made. Babies are designed to draw us in, to care for them, protect them from the world. This protective desire is present in parents, certainly, but also in the world at large. Protection of a new birth *parent* is less important in our society, and often mothers and birth parents are treated similarly to a candy wrapper tossed to the side once the treat is unwrapped. So much more than a vessel, mothers and birth parents are also deserving of care and support, and recognition of the major life shift that they are undertaking. Becoming a parent changes the way we perceive ourselves and the way we are perceived by the world. Making a major life shift is hard enough without sleep deprivation, intense hormonal changes, physical repercussions of birth, and caring for a new human being. Add those in and it's truly a wonder new parents are able to hold themselves upright!

One truly wild aspect of being postpartum is that once you leave the hospital or birth center or once the midwife leaves your home, you may not be seen again by a care provider for up to six weeks! As of 2018, the American College of Obstetricians and Gynecologists (ACOG) recognized that this was a failing of the maternal health care system. Postpartum health needs to be prioritized. ACOG now says that "postpartum care should become an ongoing process, rather than a single encounter, with services and support tailored to each woman's individual needs. It is recommended that all women have contact with their obstetrician–gynecologists or other obstetric care providers within the first three weeks postpartum." But although this suggestion has been publicized for years, it's not yet being routinely practiced by care providers. Consequently, on this side of having a baby, your sense that you aren't being cared for isn't an illusion; there's not a lot of support.

If it's possible, have a network of support in place prior to arriving on postpartum island. Your network might include friends and family, or also food delivery services, lactation consultants, pelvic health providers, a postpartum doula, postpartum support groups, a therapist, and care providers. And also, yoga: the value of attending a postpartum yoga class or workshop is that you can find safe ways to move your body *and* connect to other new moms and parents in a safe environment. If you can't find or attend an in-person postpartum yoga class, look for one online. Online postpartum classes can also create beautiful connections—we've seen that happen with the ones we've taught!

postpartum

You might find other avenues of community and support: If you are nursing or pumping human milk, lactation circles and breastfeeding cafés are another great way to find connection, support, and camaraderie during this strange, wonderful new time. Depending on which state you live in, you may not need a referral to see a pelvic care provider; you might be able to schedule that appointment on your own. And while your primary care provider might suggest you schedule your postpartum visit six weeks out from birth, consider asking if you can schedule it three to four weeks out instead. In short, the first weeks and months of your baby's life might be challenging for you, and if so, we promise that feeling is not a unique one. The shift you're undergoing is a huge one; we encourage you to seek out all the support and help you can get.

WISDOM
do I have to wait six weeks before I do yoga?

No! This is a widespread misconception that we're so happy to address. ACOG says, "If you had a healthy pregnancy and a normal vaginal delivery, you should be able to start exercising again soon after the baby is born. Usually, it is safe to begin exercising a few days after giving birth—or as soon as you feel ready. If you had a cesarean birth or complications, ask your [provider or physician] when it is safe to begin exercising again."

Gentle movement, like walking, yoga, and stretching, is a great place to begin in the early days of being postpartum. Depending on the length of your birth or the type of birth experience you had, it may feel really good to move your body. As you begin to move and explore, your body is your source of wisdom; listen to it. There is no need to overdo your effort, and there is no such thing as doing too little. Inside your uterus is a dinner plate–size wound (where your placenta was attached to the uterine wall), and even though this wound is not visible, it is very much there, and it is very much healing.

MOVE
single poses for resetting and recovery

Being postpartum brings limitations: Your body is physically recovering, you're not getting uninterrupted sleep, and your time is suddenly devoted to nurturing your baby. These poses are not necessarily meant to build up to a yoga practice although you may do them together if you have the time. If you have five minutes to yourself, we suggest choosing one of these poses and spending time getting into the pose and breathing there. All these are safe, gentle, and useful for the early days of being postpartum. You'll want two blankets, a bolster or couch cushion, and two yoga blocks for these poses.

Thread the needle

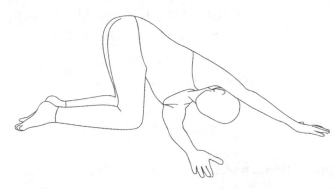

Start on your hands and knees. As you inhale, sweep your right arm upward, and as you exhale, thread it under your body, resting on your right shoulder and the right side of your head. (If your head or shoulders don't touch the floor here, add a blanket or pillow underneath.) Walk your left hand forward until your arm is stretched out long. (If you'd like, you could wrap your left arm behind your back instead. Maybe experiment to determine which one feels best.) Rest here. When you're ready, switch sides and repeat.

Cow face blanket wrap

Start seated. Cross your right leg tightly over your left, stacking your knees, so your right knee is above your left. Wrap a folded blanket around your back and hold the ends of it in your hands, pulling so that the blanket gives you a hug. You can stay seated

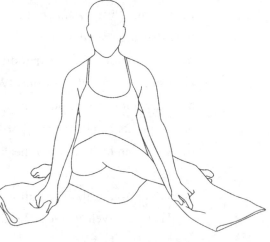

tall or lean forward over your legs. Stay for a good number of breaths, and then switch and repeat the pose with your left leg on top.

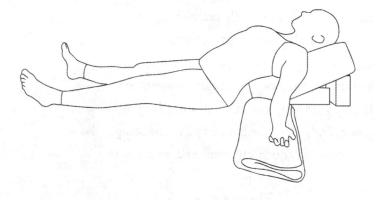

Supported fish

Set up your blocks at the end of your mat, one positioned higher than the other. Place your bolster or couch cushion on top to create a ramp. Fold your two blankets and lie back over the bolster ramp. Position the blankets under your arms, and take your arms into a T shape, so that you are able to completely release your arms, and your elbows and forearms feel supported. Stay here for as long as this pose feels good.

WISDOM
the necessity of self-kindness

In yoga and Buddhist philosophy, *ahimsa* translates to something like nonharming or compassion. Ahimsa asks us to keep others in mind and to move in the world from a place of love and nonharming. But another important way to practice ahimsa is in the most central, important relationship of your life: the one with yourself. We know right now that the relationship you have with yourself is changing, and the relationship you have with your child is expanding who you even consider yourself to be! That's why ahimsa is so crucial right now. When we practice ahimsa in relation to ourselves, we consider our self-talk, our words, and our actions in relation to us. We think about how our thoughts can be harming or healing—and we think about how the ways we move our body can be harming or healing, too!

One time, in a particularly tough, teary postpartum moment, Alexandra said to her husband, "You're always so kind to me!"

He said, "Well, you're so hard on yourself! Someone has to be."

That really stuck with her. While we want to surround ourselves with compassionate and kind loved ones, the person who should be most loving, kind, protective, and compassionate toward yourself? *You.* Does this sound familiar? As you move into motherhood and parenthood and all the choices, surprises, and shifts that it requires, we invite you to go easy on yourself and to be kind to the new being that has been born: not your child, but you. We invite you to move, breathe, and practice ahimsa—first and most important, to yourself.

Ahimsa in the context of the postpartum period may look like watching your thoughts carefully and noticing if they are judgmental or focused on your shortcomings. Ahimsa to yourself may look like reaching out for help when you need it—whether that's help doing the dishes or help with nursing (if you are choosing to nurse) or help with your mental health from a therapist.

Ahimsa to yourself during this time means that you develop love for your body as it has arrived in this new world: changed by pregnancy and birth, but still your body. And if "developing love" for your body as it is now seems impossible, then finding acceptance is a close second. Kindness to yourself in this time period means moving your body in gentle and thoughtful ways, finding patience, and taking time to rest before you dive into faster-paced yoga and movement classes. As you move into the world of being postpartum, find acceptance for your body's limitations, knowing that your body will change, rebound, shift, and grow stronger over time.

MOVE
your first yoga practice after giving birth

If you're accustomed to sun salutations and plank push-ups, this very chill, gentle practice may feel extremely mellow to you. That's the point! It's a great way to start. After more time has passed, and you feel stronger, move on to the sequences in Chapters 9 and 10. For now, take this practice as an opportunity to check in on your body and see how things feel. In all these poses, squirm, wiggle, and explore. Your first yoga practice is a time for you to listen to your body. This practice can be done in as little as ten or fifteen minutes. You don't need any props (or even a mat if you have carpeted flooring or a rug to lie on).

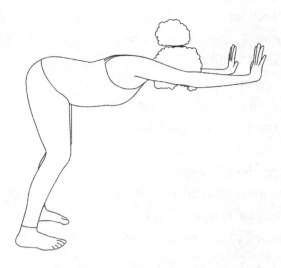

Down dog at the wall

Start by facing a blank stretch of wall. Step far enough away from the wall that you can fold forward and place your hands on the wall, making an L shape with your body. Position your hands directly out from your shoulders. Bend your knees slightly and explore gentle cat (flexion) and cow (extension) movements with your spine. You might also rock your hips from side to side, shrug your shoulders, or investigate any other movement your body wants to do. Stay here exploring and breathing for as long as you want.

Supine pelvic tilts

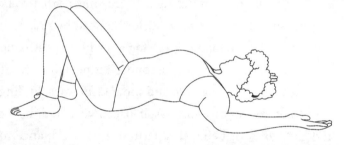

Come on to your back on the floor, bend your knees, and rest your arms next to your torso. As you inhale, let your rib cage lift and direct your tailbone downward toward the floor. You might imagine your pelvis as a bowl of water; as you breathe in, the water sloshes toward your feet. As you exhale, draw your lower back toward the floor and pull your rib cage back down into your torso. You might imagine that same bowl of water tipping back toward your belly. As you move through these pelvic tilts, you might notice slight core engagement on the exhalation. If you don't yet have that awareness, that's okay, too. It will come. You might practice five to ten rounds of these pelvic tilts.

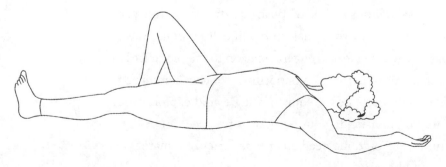

Leg slides

From your back with bent knees, inhale. As you exhale, slowly slide your right leg straight. Take your time sliding your leg out until it is fully straightened. Then, inhale again, and as you exhale, slowly re-bend your knee, sliding your foot along the floor to return to the starting position. Repeat this with your left leg sliding out and back in. You can practice this several times with each leg, if it feels comfortable.

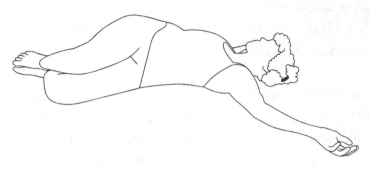

Supine twist (any variation)

From your back with bent knees, drop your knees to one side. Your arms can be in a T shape, cactus arms, or any other position that allows for a sensation of opening. If there is another variation of supine twist that you prefer (crossing the top leg over the bottom one or extending out your top leg), make adjustments to find the pose you prefer. This is a no-effort twist. Stay on the first side for as long as you'd like. Repeat, twisting to the other side.

WISDOM
vata in the postpartum period

Ayurvedic expert Melissa Ming Foynes, PhD, shares her understanding of how yoga's sister science can help us conceptualize the postpartum period. In Ayurveda, the most common element of the postpartum period is vata, a combination of air and ether. This air-and-ether heavy time period can result in a sense of discombobulation, anxiety, and creative energy.

In Ayurveda, the early postpartum time is considered a "sacred window" for the birthing person to rest, sleep, eat, get nourishment, heal, and bond with their child(ren). The expression "Forty-two days for forty-two years" conveys the sentiment that investing in nourishment during this time promotes long-term vitality and well-being for everyone in the family system. While Ayurveda has a variety of recommendations that can facilitate optimal healing and recovery and soften the transition, a systematic review of postpartum practices from fifty-one studies in

postpartum

more than twenty countries published in *Women's Health* titled, "Traditional Postpartum Practices and Rituals: A Qualitative Systematic Review," demonstrated that, cross-culturally, it is common for there to be organized support for the birthing person: periods of rest, foods that are recommended and cautioned against, and practices related to infant care and breastfeeding. Even in an "uncomplicated" birth experience, recovery time for various systems in the body can take at least three, and up to eight, weeks. Yet everyone's transition into parenthood is unique and multifaceted, and the body is only one dimension of healing.

Ayurveda teaches us about the importance of tuning in to imbalances in our bodies, minds, and hearts, and holistically working toward balance in a way that takes into account the nature of the imbalance and our *unique* constitution. I think of these imbalances as wise messages about what needs our attention most. The process of listening to and responding to these imbalances is not one that can be rushed. Like soothing a baby to sleep, it takes the time it takes.

Ayurveda teaches us about the importance of tuning in to imbalances in our bodies, minds, and hearts.

Per Ayurveda, everyone has a *vata* (a combination of the air and ether elements) imbalance postpartum, regardless of their unique constitution or how the birth unfolded. This imbalance exists because vata is the primary energy that mobilizes birth to happen and, after birth, air accumulates in the bodily cavities that the baby, placenta, and enlarged organs once occupied. Vata imbalances can lead to you feeling emotionally vulnerable, ungrounded, unfocused, anxious, worried, and can also cause constipation, memory difficulties, poor circulation, and dehydration. They can also affect the quality of human milk, the gastrointestinal health of the baby, and bonding/attachment between the baby and parent. However, some people may be more affected by these imbalances than others. For example, if someone is constitutionally high in vata, and/or had a baby during a vata time of year (late fall or winter in the northern hemisphere), their vata imbalance may be higher than someone who is constitutionally low in vata. Or, if someone had a stressful or traumatic birth experience, vata may also be higher since stress causes increased vata. While there are specific vata-pacifying recommendations for daily routines, nutrition, movement, pranayama, meditation, infant care, and so forth, not everyone's systems will respond similarly. This again requires a willingness to take a slow and thoughtful approach to observe what is and isn't working so that adaptations can be made as needed.

REFLECT
meditation that might actually just be sleep

We get that you are too tired to do anything meditative that requires much effort. Holding yourself fully upright for any prescribed period of time may feel close to impossible. We ask that you engage with this meditation completely supine and as supported as you can possibly be. If you only have a certain amount of time, set a timer, so you can relax, knowing it's okay to fall asleep. If you have all the time in the world, skip the timer. And if you fall asleep over the course of this meditation, all the better!

Adjust your body for maximum comfort and start to find the rhythm of your breathing. Close your eyes. Imagine yourself in the safest, coziest space you can. It may be that the bed you're in at the moment feels just like that, so you can tune into your surroundings without imagining anything! But likely, you might harken back to your childhood bedroom or think of a supportive hammock swinging in a summer breeze or imagine you're in an enclosed tent. Visualize whatever connotes safety, comfort, and groundedness for you. Keep adding details to your visualization: the color of your blanket, the time of day outside your cozy space, etc. If you fall asleep, fantastic. If you don't, that's okay, too; allow your body to relax into this space of security and sanctuary for as long as you can.

BREATHE
diaphragmatic breathing, with core and pelvic floor awakening

We looked at diaphragmatic breathing during the prenatal period, and this is an important breath practice during the postpartum period, too, as you reconnect to your body. Diaphragmatic breathing helps you access your core and your pelvic floor, two areas that may feel less accessible now that you have carried a baby for

postpartum

nine-plus months and gone through labor and birth. This practice can be done lying flat on your back if that's comfortable. You can have your legs straight or your knees bent. It may also be nice to prop up your pelvis and seat on a bolster, stack of pillows, or couch cushion so that you slightly elevate your lower torso.

As before, when you inhale, feel a sensation of opening in the front plane of your body: Let your belly extend outward. As you exhale, let your abdomen fall and soften. You can place your hands on your belly to keep awareness of the sensation of your breath.

As you continue this breath practice, start to notice that at the bottom of each exhalation, you can gently lift and engage your pelvic floor and, at the same time, gently draw your lower ribs closer together, to tighten and turn on the muscles of your belly space. With every breath out, pay closer attention to this core-and-pelvic-floor awakening. When you first start this breath practice postpartum, you may not be able to find those sensations of engagement. Over time, they will return.

MOVE
gentle core awareness through your day

In the diaphragmatic breathing section, you learned how to feel your pelvic floor lightly lift and your core space lightly engage as you exhaled your breath. As you move through your day, you can help your body maintain its (newfound, maybe tenuous) stability by finding this gentle bracing before you climb out of bed (remember to roll to your side first!), before you pick your baby up, before you lift anything (especially a cumbersome car seat!). It's not that your muscles aren't working—they are. Muscles fire automatically, in response to stressors we give them. But after you carry a baby in your body for forty-plus weeks, your core and pelvic floor muscles may be weaker and a little less responsive than they were previously. Being mindful and intentional in firing them up before you ask them to work is a good way to reconnect to your body and support your healing.

RELATE
sleep-deprived yoga

Erin, yoga practitioner and teacher and mom to a baby on the cusp of toddlerhood, shares the value of postpartum yoga, postpartum community, breath, and mantra on and off the mat.

Postpartum yoga offered me the opportunity to connect with other new moms, folks who were sleep-deprived like me. Folks who could tell you explicit details about the contents of their baby's diaper like I could. Folks who felt overstimulated and overwhelmed and undersupported just like I did. And what's more, postpartum yoga offered me the opportunity to connect with moms who had done all this before. Mothers who could listen and understand and validate my experience but who could also say, "What you are doing right now is really hard, but it will get better . . . maybe not easier, but better." It is a true gift (and a necessity) to be seen for the hard work that mothering requires and to be in community with other people doing that hard work.

I do not know how postpartum parents figure out newborn and baby sleep without yoga experience. Finding our breath in difficult or uncomfortable moments is what yoga helps us to practice and being able to calm your nervous system with long, slow inhales and exhales while your sweet baby wails in the middle of the night is crucial. I will never forget bouncing over and over and over again on my yoga ball while holding my infant son as he cried one night. All I could do was whisper to myself, "You can do this," a mantra I use frequently in my yoga practice. I was saying it to my son, but I was saying it to myself too.

postpartum

single poses for resetting and recovery

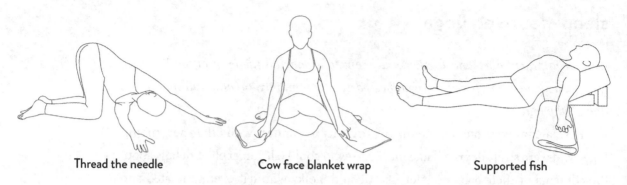

Thread the needle

Cow face blanket wrap

Supported fish

your first yoga practice after giving birth

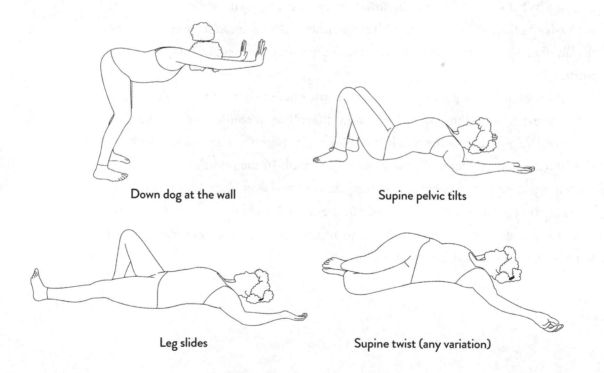

Down dog at the wall

Supine pelvic tilts

Leg slides

Supine twist (any variation)

how to breathe when you want to cry (or scream)

One in five women will deal with a perinatal mental-health concern. While we tend to be most familiar with postpartum depression and postpartum anxiety, mood disorders can manifest at any time from conception through pregnancy and into the postpartum period. Existing mood disorders can also be exacerbated by fluctuating hormones, which is why it's vital to work closely with doctors, therapists, and other care providers before, during, and after pregnancy to decide on the best means and methods of therapy for you as you navigate this huge change. Mood disorders are the single biggest hardship faced by new moms and parents of newborns.

Before we had children, we thought about postpartum depression (and the like) as a light switch: You either had it (flicked on), or you didn't (flicked off). Instead, like so many other issues of mothering and parenting, rather than black and white, postpartum mood is in the gray: There is a broad spectrum of mood issues that occur postpartum, and rarely do we see new moms who aren't *somewhere* on that spectrum. If you are feeling sad, anxious, scared, overwhelmed, or having big feelings that are out of the norm for you, you're not alone.

postpartum

Because postpartum mood issues do exist on a spectrum, different people need different things to feel whole, functional, and at peace. We have had students who wisely sought out residential facilities for postpartum treatment. Different variables may mean that your path to healing includes necessary medication and therapy.

The tools of yoga can help, too: Behavioral Activation (BA) Psychotherapy may be an important tool for perinatal depression and anxiety. In BA, new moms and birth parents are taught ways to push back against ruminating on or indulging their moods. As perinatal mood specialist Samantha Hellberg put it, "We're sad, so we listen to Adele. We're exhausted, so we channel surf." While that can feel good in the moment, she points out that "It can get us stuck in a vicious cycle where we feel down, so we withdraw and stop doing the things we enjoy or that fill our cup. BA works to create small, consistent changes to daily behavior to help us lift our moods and feel more connected to the things that give our lives joy and meaning." Within the space of simple daily changes that bring joy, we think meditation, movement, and breathwork have a place.

WISDOM
postpartum mental health and sleep

Liz Harden, MPH, sleep expert and mom of two, shares her thoughts on the connection between mental health and sleep, and what you can do in the first weeks postpartum to set you and your baby up for good sleep as you both grow.

When our sleep suffers, we suffer. Sleep supports all systems of the body and all components of healthy living. Research shows that inadequate or poor-quality sleep can increase risk for mental-health disorders such as depression, anxiety, and psychosis, both in onset and worsening of symptoms. As anyone who has had a rough night knows, we tend to feel more anxious and distressed following poor sleep.

Sleep deprivation is a fixture in those first weeks of new motherhood. Newborns sleep in thirty-minute to three-hour chunks around the clock, so you can do the math to see how much you'll be up in the night. The acute shifts in hormone levels, fatigue from giving birth, emotional stress of adjusting to your new life, and the twenty-four-hour work of caring for your newborn can lead to exhaustion. If you're experiencing fatigue and a prickly mood during the first few weeks after giving birth, you're in good company. Your sleep is suffering at a time when you need your rest the most.

There is a growing body of evidence demonstrating the relationship between poor sleep and perinatal mood disorders. The important take-home message here is that, yes, sleep will suffer in the early weeks with your newborn. But if the sleep disruption continues, you are at risk of developing a perinatal mood disorder, so let's talk about how to protect your sleep and your rest during this vulnerable time.

The important take-home message here is that, yes, sleep will suffer in the early weeks with your newborn.

Avoid overtiredness: Logic may tell you that keeping your baby awake longer will help them sleep longer. Resist this logic and embrace the powerful knowledge that avoiding overtiredness can be the difference between a baby who peacefully drifts into slumber and one who screams their head off for hours before finally conking out. Learn your baby's sleepy cues and be sure to soothe them for sleep as soon as you see a sign. Also consider writing down the maximum recommended awake times for your baby's age and aim to never cross that line, unless of course you get to know your baby and realize they truly need a little more time awake. But remember, keeping your baby awake longer before bed will not result in longer stretches of sleep at night.

Embrace the rhythm of the sun: Expose your newborn to natural light patterns like morning sunshine, high noon, sunset, and dusk. These natural light cues might not immediately synchronize newborn sleep patterns, but they will likely help. Including your newborn in your daily activities will also help to establish a clear delineation between day and night and help nudge them toward longer stretches of sleep (eventually).

Establish a bedtime routine: With a consistent bedtime routine, your baby ends the day feeling connected, secure, and ready for sleep. There's growing evidence that having a consistent bedtime routine will actually lead to better sleep. And the calming activities that foster deep connection will ensure they feel safe and secure.

Keep the night boring: Preserve the "nighttime vibe" by moving them minimally, doing what you need to do in low lighting, and putting them right back down after feedings and diaper changes.

postpartum

Set a pro-sleep environment: Keep the sleep space cool, dark, and quiet. This cave-like environment sends the message to your baby's brain: It's time for sleep. If your house isn't quiet, use white noise.

Respond mindfully to crying: If you think your baby is awake or waking up, pause, take a few deep breaths, and allow yourself to respond mindfully instead of reacting immediately. Remember that newborns spend a lot of time in active sleep and are loud as they seemingly act out their dreams. But in that active sleep state, they don't need to wake up all the way!

Enlist another caregiver to take a night shift: While it's unrealistic to expect your newborn to sleep long enough for you to wake up feeling perfectly refreshed, enlisting a co-parent, friend, or family member, or postpartum doula to take on a night shift for you can make all the difference in the world. If a few times per week you are able to get a solid three to five hour chunk of sleep at the start of the night, this will ensure that you are getting at least two full sleep cycles worth of deep sleep. And deep sleep is what our bodies need to feel restored.

Practice restorative yoga: When we can't actually sleep, restorative yoga is the next best thing.

Nap: Yes, you've heard this a billion times, but please, as much as within your ability and as circumstances allow, nap when your baby is napping. Or at least lay down in savasana.

Practice restorative yoga: When we can't actually sleep, restorative yoga is the next best thing. Restorative poses can fortify and restore you, and you can often do them with your baby in tow.

While none of these tips will automatically lead to your newborn sleeping longer stretches so that you can sleep longer stretches, taken together and practiced intentionally, you can rest assured, knowing that you are setting your baby up for the very best sleep they are capable of achieving at this young age. They will sleep the best they possibly can, and you will be better equipped to endure this period of poorer-quality rest.

BREATHE
sigh it out

A breath practice often called the "physiological sigh" can serve as a useful reset when you're feeling stressed, emotional, or overwhelmed. This breath is practiced by taking two inhalations through your nose, followed by a long exhale out of your mouth. Sighing is something our bodies do naturally and involuntarily. We often sigh as we get sleepy (a yawn is a type of sigh), or to regulate our emotions after we've cried or been otherwise upset. And even more importantly, sighing is crucial for long-term, normal lung function. When you inhale two times in a row, filling your lungs, you inflate tiny, collapsed air sacs. When you follow that by a long sigh out, you're sending a signal to your brain to slow your heart rate and a signal to your body to relax. By mindfully practicing this breath, you can offer your body the gift of stress reduction. And on the path of motherhood, stress reduction is invaluable.

Find any comfortable seat, or you can even practice this breath standing. If possible, close your eyes. Inhale through your nose, until your lungs are almost full. Then, in quick succession, inhale again, "topping off" your breath. Follow this by exhaling through your mouth *slowly*, taking your time. Repeat this up to three times or until you feel a little more present, calm, and grounded.

WISDOM
contentment as a radical practice

The Sanskrit word *santosha* means contentment. In yoga philosophy, santosha is one of the *niyamas*—the principles of personal observance that yoga practitioners try to follow. It's situated around other principles that mean devotion to the yoga practice, cleanliness, self-study, and surrender to the divine. Out of all these, radical contentment—accepting and loving the life you have right now—might be the hardest. The harder we seek it, or think of it as happiness, the more elusive it can be. In reality, it actually means to be fully with whatever it is that we're feeling—be that sadness, boredom, angst, or anger. Contentment is to bring an open heart and

postpartum

acceptance to the moment, to be present with what is. Discontentment is really just the idea that there can be anything else in any given moment—it just isn't possible.

Lauren has a beloved family in her life she's been connected to for many years. She used to babysit for the kids when she was in college, and clearly remembers when her friend, the children's mom, then in her forties, said that she had *just* realized that she was living her life—actually living it. Lauren, now in her forties, has been struck by that time and again during her children's younger years. There's a saying: "People are always *getting ready* to live." It can come as a stark realization that we're actually living our lives now.

It's a radical act to be okay with that life, even with the hardship and challenge it entails. It is easy enough to be content with life when we're feeling happy and well rested. It's a kind of rebellion against our culture to be teary and tired, with sore nipples and a new, changed body, and to still recognize that *this* life is exactly where you are and to sit with that, fully accepting the moment.

REFLECT
the ocean refuses no river

One of our favorite chants is this refrain: *The ocean refuses no river*. Attributed to Sufi mystics, we first heard it from yoga teacher Kristin Cooper-Gulak, founder of Kunga Yoga.

This chant can feel like a call for body love and self-love, amidst all the swirling emotions of being postpartum. This chant can feel like a reminder that the divine source is one of all-encompassing acceptance: All are received and welcomed. This chant helps you recall the central truth that there is nothing you have to do, fix, or change. You are worthy as you are: The ocean refuses no river. In this new landscape of emotions, mood, and motherhood, remembering your worth is vital.

WISDOM
a postpartum doula for support

Quanisha Callwood, MSW, CLC, discusses the role of a postpartum doula and the support inherent in this work.

Postpartum doula work is an invaluable offering for new families. The postpartum period is full of many transitions, and without support, many of those transitions can become traumas. It is during the postpartum period that we are seeing many issues arise, including perinatal mood and anxiety disorders. I've always been so concerned with the lack of support during the postpartum period, and because of this, I provide services that focus on major aspects of after-birth care.

During the postpartum period, I meet with families forty-eight to seventy-two hours after birth. During this visit, I tend to the needs of the family. This can include infant care, allowing mom or birth parent an opportunity to shower, or spend some time alone. I inquire about their adjustment to this new life and listen. The most popular service I provide is overnight support. During this time, I allow the birthing parent the time needed to rest and heal. I assure my families that it is my duty during this time to create a comforting space for them to rest and within that, I want them to also be assured that their baby is in the best care. Newborn/infant care is such a large part of this overnight support, and I am always overjoyed by the refreshed faces I witness in the morning.

REFLECT
the easiest baby book

The sense that you're failing at motherhood or somehow not doing all the things you envisioned could exacerbate challenging postpartum emotions. Lauren had a vision of keeping a detailed account of her days, all baby pictures organized, and went out and purchased a baby keepsake book at Hallmark when her son, Simon, was three weeks old. Simon is now eleven. His baby book ends at three months. All of us make grand plans and sometimes it is best to know when to let those go.

postpartum

Instead of keeping careful track of how many naps your baby was taking at the six-week mark, who came to visit, and what the most popular movie was on the day of their birth, you might try keeping an e-mail journal instead. When poignant, or cute, or landmark moments happen in her daughter's life, Alexandra will send her daughter a quick e-mail (to an e-mail address she set up in her daughter's name that she will one day be able to access) and describe the moment, almost in real time. Sometimes she includes pictures and videos. It's quick and easy and very accessible—and it's done.

MOVE
mood boost yoga

If you don't want to move, guess what? You don't have to! But here's a practice that invites you to quickly flow, breathe, and expand your body in ways that may remind you that you are a radiant, vibrant being—even if you haven't showered in a while, and you're running on coffee and two hours of sleep. Let this be a messy flow, and for the last two poses, set up near a wall, so you can put a hand on the wall for balance. None of these movements should feel like they need to be precise or that they need to be repeated a certain number of times. There is no goal for whether your arms are straight or whether your leg is in a certain position; there is no focus on or concern for alignment. Just move, play, and experience your body and your breath. This is a good practice if you feel sad or anxious, or if you're just not sure what you feel. You don't even need a mat for this.

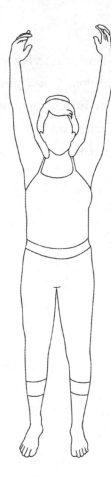

Breath of joy start

Start standing with your knees slightly bent. Inhale briefly and sweep your arms overhead. Inhale briefly again to sweep your arms back downward. Inhale fully and completely as you sweep your arms overhead once more.

Breath of joy finish

From a full inhale with your arms overhead, sweep your arms downward, and fold at the waist (how far you fold is up to you). As you do this part of the breath of joy, exhale out through your mouth making a "hah" sound.

Repeat these breaths and movements until you feel more invigorated, lighter, and more present.

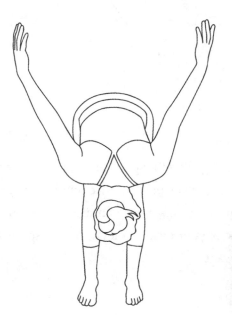

postpartum

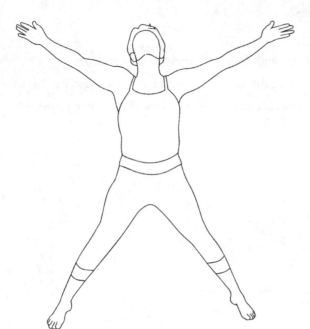

Standing star

From standing, take your feet as wide as feels good and reach your arms out and into a T or Y position. Inhale, and as you exhale imagine you are radiating energy out of your arms and legs—feel your spirit expand, even as you remain in stillness.

Warrior 3 kick flow (standing)

Set up standing parallel to a wall. Place your hand on the closest wall, so you have balance support. Your other hand can be at your heart or hip, or you can stretch this arm overhead. As you inhale, kick your outer leg forward into space, lifting to any degree you want.

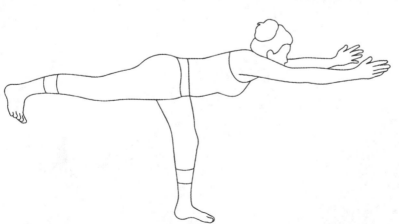

Warrior 3 kick flow

From the position of one leg kicked forward, transition that leg behind you on the exhale, moving into a Warrior 3 shape.

Your free hand can remain at your heart or hip, or you can extend your arm back toward your hips.

Repeat these two shapes several times on each side if it feels good to do so. Then, switch sides and repeat this little flow. If you revisit this sequence over time, you can transition away from a wall and add in full balance.

WISDOM
the push and pull

One of our favorite motherhood cartoons shows two panels. In the first, a haggard and exhausted mother is frantically soothing her baby, thinking, *Please just go to sleep!* And in the second panel, the baby is asleep in a crib in the background, and the mom is now in bed, looking at pictures on her phone of her smiling and sweet baby thinking, *Oh, I miss her now!*

This captures the absolute ambivalence of motherhood: the pull of both wanting to be there every moment, and the desperation of wanting a moment to yourself. This push and pull is nearly a universal experience; you're suddenly the support person for the neediest little being, so of course there are moments when you'll feel deep resistance to this ceaseless role. Not every moment of parenting a baby is a rewarding, fulfilling experience, and moving away from having full control over your time and your life can be a cause for mourning.

In yoga philosophy, *raga* and *dvesha* are two of the *kleshas* (causes of suffering). Commonly translated as attachment (raga) and aversion (dvesha), they are very much two sides of the same coin. The solution is awareness: to notice when you feel overly attached to the point of anxiousness, and to notice when you feel overwhelmed and averse and need a break.

Ultimately, though, wrestling with attachment and aversion—sometimes to the same things or for the same experiences—is not just a common experience of motherhood, but a common experience of humanity. If you find yourself irrationally attached to your child or if you find yourself deeply averse to moments with your child, know that these are both normal. And with time and reflection, the grip of raga and dvesha will lessen.

postpartum

BREATHE
breath regulation for mood regulation

Exploring holding the breath at the top of an inhale (*kumbhaka antara*) or at the bottom of the exhale (*kumbhaka bahya*) are both nice ways to calm the body down and feel a little more centered and grounded. During these tumultuous early days, anything that can help stabilize your mood is probably welcome. To practice kumbhaka antara, take in a big belly breath. Hold your breath without moving into a space of discomfort. Then, slowly release your breath, taking your time. The goal is not to strain but to find stillness in the brief cessation of the breath.

To practice kumbhaka bahya, breathe out completely and then hold, waiting until you feel compelled to breathe again (but don't wait until you're gasping!). Then inhale and exhale slowly and repeat.

REFLECT
feel your feelings

In her book, *Operating Instructions*, Anne Lamott details the landmarks and minutiae of her son's first year. After being a parent for three weeks, Lamott comments on four other friends who have recently given birth saying, "I do not believe any of them are having these awful thoughts. One of the worst things about being a parent, for me, is the self-discovery, the being face-to-face with one's secret insanity and brokenness and rage." Becoming a parent is hard, regardless of how beautiful and wonderful it is, and our feelings are exacerbated by lack of sleep and seismic hormonal shifts. Lauren still remembers the rage she would feel with her innocent newborn son when she'd gently be putting him back to sleep after nursing and rocking him, only to have a full-on diaper blowout the minute she set him down. We all have moments in parenting when we confront despair and anger, fear and loneliness. Acknowledging the ambivalence through mantra can be one way to help normalize the feelings that you're experiencing. Below are a few of our favorites:

It's okay to feel this way.
I'm doing my best.
I forgive myself.
This is really hard.
I'm not alone.
I can ask for help.
I am not my thoughts.
I can take a step back.
I can breathe right now.
This experience does not define motherhood.
This moment does not define me as a mom.

postpartum

mood boost yoga

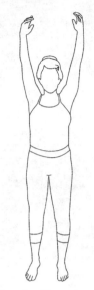

Breath of joy start

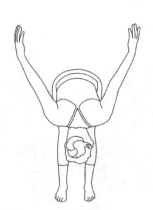

Breath of joy finish

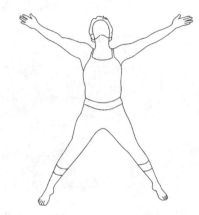

Standing star

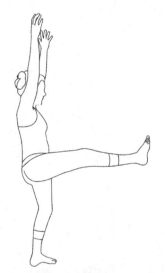

Warrior 3 kick flow (standing)

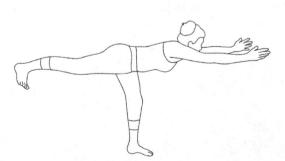

Warrior 3 kick flow

Chapter Ten

postpartum poses—the good, the bad, and the less attractive

As you settle into being a new mom or birth parent in this postpartum stage, your desire to move your body safely may increase. The discussion around being postpartum tends to split into two: People either focus on shifting out of this period as rapidly as possible (that "get your body back" nonsense we discussed in Chapter 8), or they lament that their body is "ruined" or "destroyed" by pregnancy and birth. The truth is that your body is *healing*. It's gone through something metamorphic, and there is a reframing and a rebirth that has to happen on this side of pregnancy.

Many of the postpartum body changes require something that you can't force: time. Healing doesn't happen overnight, and recovery takes time. You're also healing and recovering while getting less sleep and being more "on" all the time. It's no wonder that you may not feel like yourself or recognize your body in the mirror.

postpartum

As you start to move, attend more yoga classes, walk, run, or return to your other previous movement modalities, there's not a lot on the "Don't do this!" list, but there are a few things you may want to avoid for a little while, and there may be a few things you want to do more of to help your body build strength in key areas.

It's helpful to avoid movements that create intra-abdominal pressure. Because all pregnant people experience *diastasis recti* (DR), a gap in the linea alba connective tissue between the muscles of the rectus abdominis (six-pack muscles), postpartum, it's wise to avoid crunches, crunch-like movements, and any movements that cause loss of integration of the core muscles. (Consider that even sitting up in bed is a crunch-like movement; during the exhausting early days of being postpartum, try to remember to roll to one side, and use your hands to support you to sit up.) If you feel like your belly is distending in any pose or exercise, skip the movement. That may mean leaving out twists in challenging poses (like revolved crescent lunge) and deep backbends (like upward-facing bow) for a while. Those types of poses put a lot of pressure on the belly space during a time when the muscles of that space need to integrate, reconnect, and heal. You may recover from any pregnancy-related DR within the first six weeks of being postpartum. But some postpartum people continue to have DR for months after pregnancy and may require support from a pelvic health provider to heal it. While your doctor or midwife may check you for a diastasis at a postpartum appointment, you can also check yourself: DR self-check tutorials abound online. But the wisest choice is to seek out pelvic health care postpartum where you will be checked for DR and other issues by an expert in the field. Norah Whitten, our friend and pelvic floor physical therapist, says, "Every woman should have at least an assessment with a pelvic health care provider postpartum so that they can ensure their pelvic floor is healing and functioning well." This is the case whether an OB or midwife cleared you, whether you had a vaginal or cesarean birth. As Whitten notes, pelvic floor therapists "help people with a number of issues during the rehab process, from pain and symptom management to rebuilding strength, and everything in between."

It's wise to avoid crunches, crunch-like movements, and any movements that cause loss of integration of the core muscles.

Your yoga practice before and during pregnancy may have been focused on expanding, stretching, opening, and building flexibility. In the postpartum period, pivot to contracting, healing, pulling inward, and building strength. That will mean focusing on dynamic movements for your hips and seat: things like active bridge pose, variations on squat, and inner-thigh and outer-hip strengtheners are useful during this time period. Try placing a block between your thighs in various poses and focus on squeezing into the midline of your body, firing up your inner thighs, pelvic floor, seat, and core.

You may notice that your upper body is tight, and your shoulders get rounder: you're suddenly carrying and feeding an eight- to twenty-pound baby in the front plane of your body all the time. To combat this, gravitate to poses that open the front of your chest (like cobra or supported fish), and that strengthen your upper back (like downward-facing dog).

Simple core engagement (not crunches!) that builds over time will help you gain strength gently. Skip boat pose, and focus instead on bird dog, supported side plank, and other shapes that help you notice your core area without exhausting it. Do a little to start, and gradually add duration and intensity.

The key to postpartum movement (like prenatal movement) is adaptability: If you're having wrist issues, choose to come into poses on your fists or forearms. If you're having any pelvic girdle pain, skip movements that exacerbate that discomfort. If you're not sure what you're feeling, go slower and let your movement practice focus on inquiry.

We've already discussed the lack of medical care for the postpartum period. But another aspect of this period that surprised us is how much people *don't* discuss. It's not just your doctors who aren't leaning into this time period; culturally, we don't sit with or honor or share about the postpartum experience. There are a lot of postpartum changes no one prepares you for or talks about, which we'll address next. But ultimately, it's helpful to know that your body will grow stronger and more familiar with time. Right now, you're in recovery.

postpartum

WISDOM
common postpartum changes

During the early postpartum period, you will likely experience *lochia* (blood and mucus from the vagina) whether you had a vaginal or cesarean birth. While this usually ends two to six weeks postpartum, there are other changes that take longer. If you tore during your child's birth, you may have stitches that are healing in your perineal area. Whether you tore or not, you may feel tender in that area, as it's done a lot of work! You might have tailbone pain (*coccydynia*) or bruising from the delivery. If you had a cesarean birth, you may experience itching and scar pain at the surgery site, and it can take up to eighteen months to fully heal. It's common to have hemorrhoids postpartum; baby weight and pushing are the culprit. As you may notice in a yoga class when you go to lift a leg in downward-facing dog, vaginal flatulence is common postpartum, as your vaginal canal is not a smooth muscle; it has pockets that get opened up through delivery and may more easily capture air afterward. (The good news is that it's normal and not an indication that anything is wrong. It will go away over time or with the support of a pelvic health professional.) As you feel stronger and more healed, exploring gentle awareness and engagement in the pelvic-floor area can help you reconnect to this space in your body.

Your hips may feel different, and they may even be slightly wider from the weight of carrying your baby and your delivery. We already talked about the possibility of diastasis recti, but even if you don't have DR, you may have a lack of core muscle sensation. If you nurse, pump, or breastfeed, you may feel a heaviness in your upper body, and your breasts may feel sensitive. We often hear about wrist issues in postpartum yoga classes. *De Quervain's tenosynovitis or radial styloid tenosynovitis* is a painful condition that affects the thumb-side wrist tendons that occurs from chronic overuse, like the motion required for lifting a baby.

Our colleague Mary Reddinger, an expert prenatal and postpartum yoga teacher, describes more changes of the postpartum period succinctly:

Think about it: while you were pregnant, your body began to compensate in order to offset the weight of your growing baby.

Your ribs expanded to make more room for your uterus, which made your diaphragm flatten out and your breath become shallow. Shallow breathing reduces your rib cage mobility (hello, neck and shoulder pain).

Your abdominal muscles and tissue stretched and thinned to make more room for your uterus—and your ribs flared, which decreased your core stability.

When your core stability decreased, other muscles figured out how to do the work of the core. Your back muscles might have taken over (hello, low back pain), or your pelvic floor muscles took over (hello, pelvic floor dysfunction). Or smaller muscles took over, leading to posture changes that decrease your glutes (hello hip pain, back pain, and flat butt).

And while we spoke on this in previous chapters, it's worth remembering that the largest changes may not be visible: postpartum mood disorder is the *most common* complication of childbirth.

If this list feels overwhelming, keep in mind that these changes happened over the course of many months, and it may take just as many months to heal.

Keep in mind that these changes happened over the course of many months, and it may take just as many months to heal.

MOVE
postpartum modifications

As you start to make your way in the world again, that may include attending classes, walking, and moving your body in ways that feel good. Thankfully, there aren't many shapes, movements, or poses that need to be avoided, but these two modifications are useful in a yoga practice or in your daily life. Both modifications give you a chance to avoid crunching or crunch-type movements that are less helpful during the healing postpartum period.

postpartum

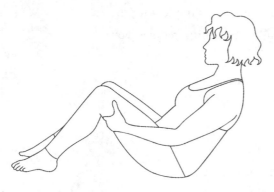

Boat modification

If you attend a yoga class and boat pose is offered, here's a good way to modify it. Keep your feet on the ground rather than lifting them up. Bring your hands to the backs of your thighs so that you are fully in control of how much work your core is doing. Allow your arms to help. Lean back, just until you feel a gentle core awakening. Stay focused on pulling in: draw your rib cage down and in, and pull the sides of your ribs inward toward each other. Imagine someone is about to tickle you or touch your belly, and brace for this. As you exhale, feel that bracing sensation tighten.

Roll to the side to sit up

When you're lying down, rather than roll up to sitting, avoid crunching your body by bending your knees, rolling to one side, and using your hands to help you press the floor away. You may be familiar with this, as it's a common way yoga teachers cue their students to exit savasana. Use this in bed, in yoga class, and anytime you are getting up from lying down.

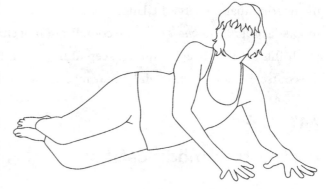

REFLECT
chanting peace

In Sanskrit, the word *shanti* means peace. While there are moments of peace in the early postpartum days, sometimes it can feel as though chaos reigns. A former student of Lauren's once bought her a mug with a fairly common quote that read, "Peace. It does not mean to be in a place where there is no noise, trouble, or hard work. It means to be in the midst of all of those things and still be calm in your heart." There are times when throwing the coffee mug across the room might be more satisfying. Most of the time, however, these words serve as a good reminder. Whether it's at the end of a yoga practice, at the start of the day, when your newborn is crying, or when you're up (again) to feed your baby in the middle of the night, chanting, repeating, or thinking this one-word mantra (*shanti*) can also serve as a helpful reminder that you can't look externally for a sense of calm and contentment. You can turn to our website for a common way of chanting shanti, or you can make up a rhythm and tune that resonates with you.

MOVE
yoga for shoulders and upper back

Postpartum, rounded shoulders are common. Alexandra remembers noticing her *kyphotic* shoulders in the mirror with horror when her daughter was just a few months old. The good news is that this can be remedied and helped with movement and exercise. This sequence offers movements to open your chest and shoulders and movements to strengthen your upper back as an antidote to this common rounding. The only prop you need for this sequence is the wall.

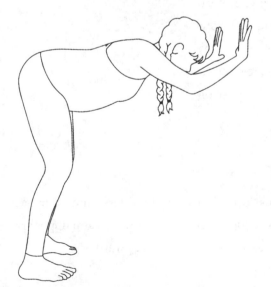

Down-dog wall push-up
Stand facing the wall. Place your hands on the wall and walk away from the wall until your body is making an L shape and your hands are parallel to your shoulders. Slightly bend your knees. As you inhale, bend your elbows, bringing your head closer to the wall, and then exhale as you push the wall away, straighten your arms, and squeeze your shoulder blades together. Repeat this until you feel reasonably fatigued.

postpartum

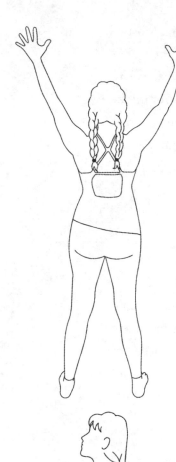

Wall hang

Stand facing the wall, then place your arms onto the wall, stretched out overhead and wider than shoulder-distance apart. Step back far enough that you can lean your head onto the wall. This can be the pose, or as you exhale, you may press your hands into and downward on the wall, as if you were hanging off the edge of a cliff and trying to pull yourself back up—which engages the muscles throughout your back.

Wall arm stretch

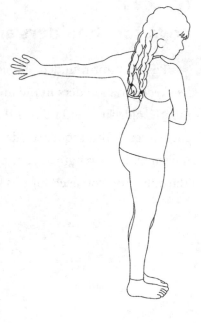

Stand parallel to the wall and sweep your arm closest to the wall along it, so that you begin to stretch your chest. Take your free arm and wrap it around the front of your body to capture your ribs and gently pull your rib cage forward. You might tip your head away from the wall and tuck your chin to find a neck stretch. Stay here until the first side feels complete, and then repeat this pose on the second side.

Wall camel

Stand at the wall with your back to it. Roll your shoulders onto your back, clasping your hands together at your seat. Lean your shoulders and upper arms into the wall and press against it as you lift your chest upward.

BREATHE
open-mouthed sighing

This breath is deceptively simple for how good it feels: Take a deep breath in through your nose, fill your lungs, and sigh out, allowing sound to occur. Repeating this breath three times might offer the most relief from tension, stress, and anxiety. You can play with adding breath retention to the top of the inhale, if it feels good to hold a moment before you sigh out. The key, though, is to allow this breath to become auditory: Make a little noise on your sigh. Sigh out in relief and surrender.

MOVE
yoga for wrists

De Quervain's tenosynovitis and other wrist issues can show up postpartum, since you're constantly lifting your baby and using your wrists. While yoga may be useful, resting or immobilizing your affected wrist (like with a compression bandage), icing, and an anti-inflammatory medication like ibuprofen may be helpful, too.

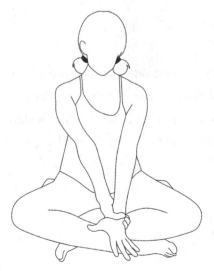

Pull your wrist

From a seated position (on the floor or in a chair), extend one arm forward. Use your other hand to grasp your extended wrist and pull your hand, creating traction and space. Repeat on the other hand.

postpartum

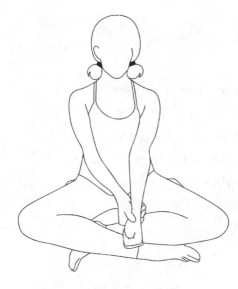

Fist stretch

Extend one arm outward, creating a fist. With your other hand, use your thumb to gently massage a line from your wrist to your thumb. Repeat on the other hand.

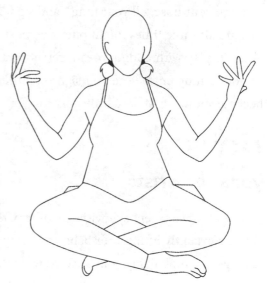

Hand shaking

Bend your elbows and shake your hands, allowing your fingers to fling through space. You can do this gently or with some vigor.

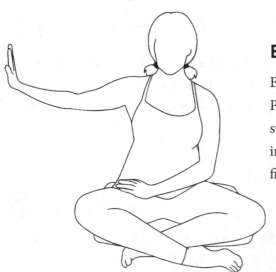

Extension hand

Extend your arm out to your side, parallel to the floor. Point your fingers at the ceiling as if you were making a stop gesture with your extended hand. Explore widening the space between your fingers and stretching your fingers outward.

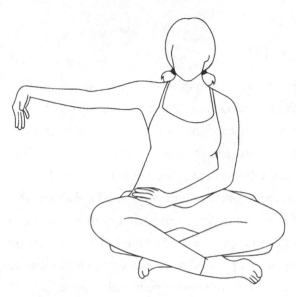

Flexion hand

Extend your arm out to your side, parallel to the floor. Point your fingers downward or curl your fingers toward the inside of your wrist. Try wiggling your fingers as if you were playing keys on a piano.

Repeat these last two poses with your second hand.

MOVE
yoga for your pelvic floor

Connecting with your pelvic floor muscles after birth can feel intimidating. The following exercise expands on the idea of diaphragmatic breathing and serves as a great way to reconnect with and strengthen this area of your body. Practice this in any position that feels comfortable and allows you to draw your awareness to your pelvis. Close your eyes and take a few deep and relaxed belly breaths. Pretend that you're taking your pelvic floor muscles up to a third-floor apartment, fortunately one with an elevator. Inhale, and as you exhale, gently and lightly draw your pelvic floor inward and upward, as if the elevator were moving from the basement to the first floor. Inhale again, and on the next exhale, engage inward and upward with slightly more vigor, visualizing the elevator moving to the second floor. Finally, inhale, and on the exhale, engage completely, drawing the elevator to the highest floor, the third-floor penthouse. Try to maintain that hold for a few rounds of breath. Then, allow the elevator to return, floor by floor, to the basement. This part may feel more challenging or more tenuous. Know that there is no success or failure here; you're exploring and feeling.

postpartum

REFLECT
love your body (or at least respect it!)

If you grew up in a Western culture as a woman, it's sort of impossible not to move into adulthood with some level of body perception issue. We are constantly bombarded with the message that our body as it is is not enough: It needs to be sexier, thinner, younger. (Ugh.) And unfortunately, a lot of the imagery of yoga (tall and lanky white women with their legs behind their heads) reinforces the idea that how your body looks or what your body can do for others is directly linked to how you should feel about your body. This culturally encouraged and long-simmering body anxiety can rear its head in the postpartum period. Working with a therapist can be helpful. But acknowledging that your feelings about your body may be complicated by these external forces can be helpful too. These reflection prompts ask you to conceive of your body from a space of love. And if loving your body feels like an impossible leap right now, you can at least respect it and the tremendous experience you just went through.

Here are the reasons I respect my body as it is right now:

As it heals, I can tell that my body needs:

If I feel negative body thoughts overwhelm me, here are some things I can do:

MOVE
yoga for core strength reconnection

Your belly has done a lot of work for the past nine-plus months, and your goal now is to gently engage the muscles that have kindly supported and birthed your baby. Reconnecting with your abdominal area might help any lower-back discomfort you've been feeling, and it may allow you to find more ease in movements like getting up from standing while holding a baby in your arms. You might try one or two of the poses offered here the first time you visit this sequence and gradually add in more. Alexandra teaches Pilates in addition to yoga, and when she came back from maternity leave, these were the poses that best prepared her to return to teaching core work!

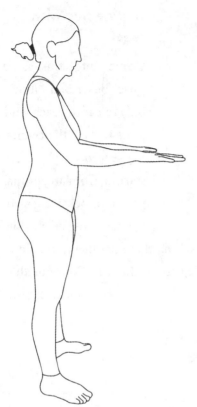

Standing core press

Stand facing a counter, the back of your couch or anywhere else where you can rest your hands on a shelf. Inhale. As you exhale, gently press into the shelf with your hands and as you do, focus on tightening and engaging the muscles of your core space. Draw your lowest ribs deeper into your body and brace your core by tightening the deepest muscle layer of your abdomen. (If this feels inaccessible to you, imagine you are preparing your body to be tickled, which can help fire up and turn on these muscles.) Practice this, inhaling to release and exhaling to reengage five or more times.

Supine bug hold

Come onto your back. Bring your knees directly above your hips with your shins parallel to the floor. Hold on to the backs of your legs with your hands, so you can offer your body support and control the level of challenge. Inhale, and as you exhale, draw your low back down toward the floor, bracing your core space. Try to hold on to that engagement as you breathe here. If this feels too easy, you can release the hold on your legs.

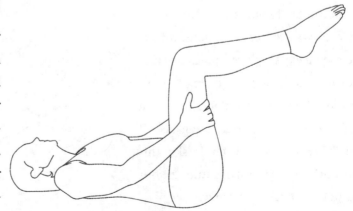

Through this pose and the ones that follow, leave the back of your head resting on the floor.

postpartum

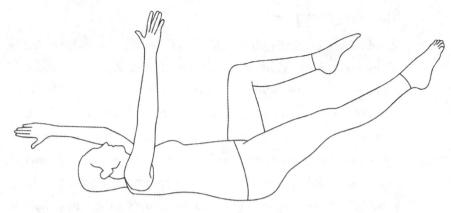

Supine bug with reach

Come into the same pose described above, only this time reach your arms toward the ceiling. Pause to be sure you are starting from an optimal position: belly engaged, rib cage tucked in, low abdominals firing. Inhale and extend your right leg and left arm, reaching them parallel to the floor. Exhale and return to the starting pose. Repeat, extending your left leg and right arm. Continue this, switching sides and exhaling to return to the starting shape, and optimal core engagement, each time.

Supine leg press

Come into the same pose described above, only this time bring your hands to the fronts of your legs, resting them between your knees and quads. Inhale, and as you exhale press your hands into your legs as if you were trying to push your feet down onto the floor. Resist that press by keeping your core engaged. If your belly domes or distends, skip this one until you are further along your postpartum healing journey.

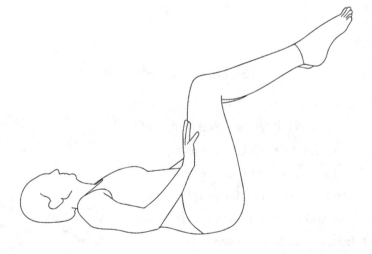

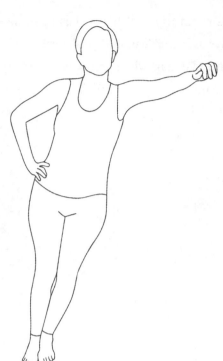

Wall side plank

Stand with feet parallel to a wall and walk your feet away from it until you can lean against the wall, resting on your forearm. For more challenge, walk farther from the wall. For more ease, move closer to it. Maintain a long line of your body, and stay focused on keeping your core engaged.

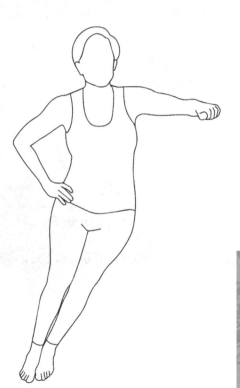

Wall side plank dip

From wall side plank, inhale to dip your hips toward the wall, and then exhale to return to the starting side plank pose. Move slowly and with control.

Repeat the last two poses on the second side.

REFLECT
mantra for motherhood

Mantra can also serve a role for parents who might find a phrase helpful to keep them present and calm, especially in the face of exhaustion, emotional changes, boredom, or anger. Our children intuitively know that repetition of phrases is one way to effect change: Consider that babies and toddlers may repeat their desires over and over. Repeating phrases out loud or in your head can help you in the hardest

postpartum

moments: at 2 A.M. heading back into your baby's room to meet their needs in some
ways, in the grocery store, when your little one has a diaper leak and you're short on
time, on the day your baby decides to skip their midday nap when *you* really needed
that nap for your mental wellness. Here are some mantras we love for those moments:

Yes, thanks.
No victims, just volunteers.
I can do things that are hard.
Teach me about kindness.
Even now, peace.

postpartum modifications

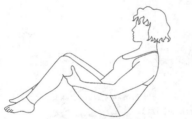

Boat modification

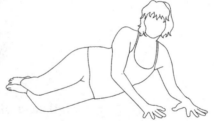

Roll to the side to sit up

yoga for shoulders and upper back

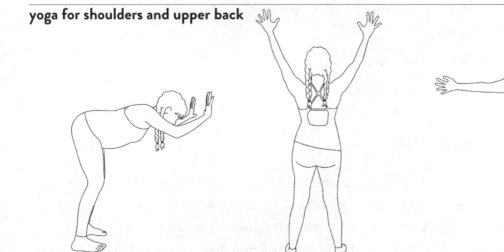

Down-dog wall push-up   Wall hang   Wall arm stretch

yoga for shoulders and upper back (continued)

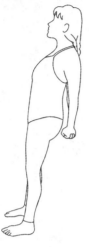

Wall camel

yoga for wrists

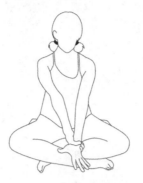

Pull your wrist

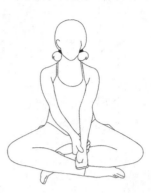

Fist stretch

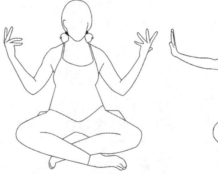

Hand shaking

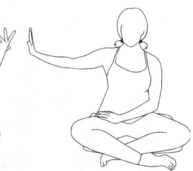

Extension hand

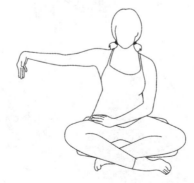

Flexion hand

yoga for core strength reconnection

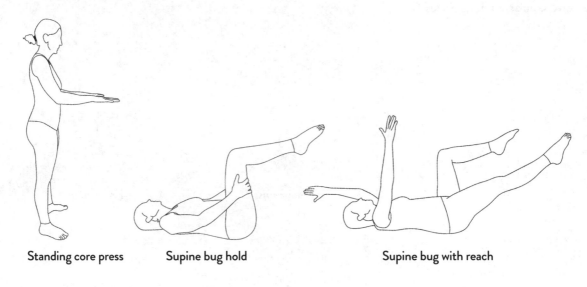

Standing core press   Supine bug hold   Supine bug with reach

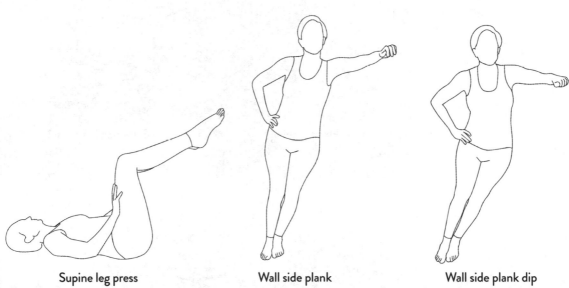

Supine leg press   Wall side plank   Wall side plank dip

Part Five

parenting

Chapter Eleven

yoga through the years

Some mornings we wake up tired, cranky, and just sort of down. It would be awesome to stumble out of bed, Disney-princess moms, moving at full tilt (fueled by zest for life rather than caffeine), full of energy, love, and unending patience for crumbs and toys everywhere. But the truth is that we are human, and sometimes we don't feel so great.

Sometimes, it's important to give energy and attention to our harder emotions. They clue us in on something that we're noticing intuitively that needs action or healing or attention. But sometimes our harder emotions are just the product of a lack of sleep, too much sugar, not enough water, a need for some movement, or alone time, and so forth and so on. Yet even though both positive and negative emotions are often fleeting, we tend to identify with those emotions. We don't just *feel* angry. We think (or say), "I *am* angry!" Yoga reminds us that our true Self is not the shifting landscape of emotions, but the rock-solid, unchanging foundation under it all. And that Self is not anger or joy or sadness or glee. That Self is just the *Self*.

As motherhood feels less new and more familiar, you might reflect on the limitations of yoga. Blasphemy, we know! But let us explain: If you are a longtime yoga practitioner, you may have been called to yoga in your twenties or thirties or even before that. Starting yoga, you may have felt an immediate difference in your mood and your physical flexibility and strength. Moving in your body may have helped you process important life experiences and helped you come to terms with some of the challenges of your youth. Yoga may have felt like a revelation! This story is not uncommon: Both of us have similar yoga stories, and so do many of our yoga colleagues. Yoga is powerful, powerful medicine.

But there was also a time later in life and further down our yoga paths when we added motherhood into our life's roles. And motherhood changed our yoga practice.

Alexandra remembers starting to feel like she was failing at yoga because it wasn't "working" as well to resolve all her stress: Her thought process started to be something like this: *Okay, if I get up early and meditate and practice, then I'll feel better. If I go to this class weekly, I'll feel better. If I commit to my handstand practice, I'll feel better.*

For Lauren, yoga felt like just one more to-do in a never-ending list—committing to a regular practice felt close to impossible given the newfound responsibilities and shift in priorities. When she got on her mat at home, no number of sun salutations could sufficiently immerse her in the present enough to forget the duties her partner was taking on in order for her to practice, the chaos of her house, or her seemingly endless exhaustion.

Inevitably, we all do feel better when we meditate and practice yoga regularly, but it helps whenever we can make the space and time for it. No amount of meditation or breathwork or movement is going to resolve all the existential crises and fears that arise with modern-day motherhood. Modern-day life is tough stuff, and there is suffering here, even for those of us with deep privilege. Also, many of the ancient yogis were ascetic men with no families. Arguably, their sphere of concern was smaller and less personal than loved ones, children, workplaces, and family. Maybe yoga solved for them things that are now far more complicated, challenging, and multifaceted in the modern, technological world.

Yoga helps you find calm, clarity, and presence.

Yoga is one important piece of your wellness on the motherhood journey. Yoga helps you find calm, clarity, and presence. It helps you remember who you are, and move away from all the noise of emotions. It's powerful, powerful medicine. It's just not the *only* medicine you may need in the challenging, stressful times of parenting. It doesn't fix things or solve things; it just gives you a chance to see things as they are, to be present to what is so that you can find the other pieces you need to fix and solve.

This is especially the case when you have young babies, toddlers, and preschoolers: Those children need physical care and presence on a scale that can be unspeakably exhausting. Along with yoga, another piece of the wellness puzzle is compassion and self-compassion. Compassion in parenting is important because it reduces suffering: yours and your children's. And ultimately, that's the point of yoga.

RELATE
the motherhood perspective shift

Sage Rountree, PhD, yoga teacher, author, and studio owner, and mother of two now-grown women, twenty-two and twenty, shares insight on how our relationship to yoga has one variable: ourselves.

While I now own a yoga studio and direct teacher trainings, my relationship with yoga got off to a rocky start. Feeling confident in my flexibility, I went to the yoga class at the gym—the one that seemed "easy" from my view on the stair-climbing machine. It was not easy! It was hard, humbling, and foreign. I had such a negative reaction that I forced myself to return the next week hoping for a better outcome.

No such luck. In my second class, the original teacher was away, and we had a substitute. She had us do partner yoga—*yuck*! I had to touch a stranger's feet! I was thoroughly done with yoga and wouldn't return for several years.

Until, expecting my first child, I went to a prenatal yoga class with my best friend and neighbor, who was also pregnant. We were happy before the class even began, chatting with our sweet classmates about how things were going. When the teacher came in, I realized it was the sub from my second-ever yoga class. But she was also pregnant, and when the time came to do partner yoga and rub each other's swollen ankles, I found I loved it. That third class marked the start of a regular practice I've had for over two decades.

What changed? It wasn't yoga. It wasn't even the teacher—she was the same woman. *It was me.* I was in a different space, physically, mentally, and spiritually.

My body was ready for the gentle level of asana we practiced. My head was ready for connection. And my heart was wide-open and humble with the recognition that the journey I was embarking on depended on the community around me.

This perspective shift was a valuable lesson that has served me well through pregnancy, parenting, and now empty nesting: Things change over time. Just because something doesn't suit the current moment doesn't mean it won't suit the very next moment, or the one after that. Just like an experience in a pose or a parenting challenge can evolve breath to breath, so can your relationship to what is happening now.

MOVE
baby and me yoga

One important way to continue your movement practice when you're exhausted and busy is to invite your baby into it! These poses are just a few examples of the ways you can add your baby into the yoga mix. In some of these, your little one gets to enjoy movement with you, and in some of these, your baby gets to watch you from a new perspective. As you try these shapes and poses, add in cuddles, tickles, kisses, and coos. Use these few poses as a jumping-off point for the other ways your sweet little one can join in your practice.

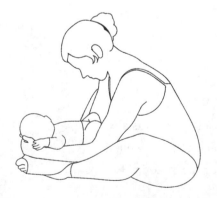

Cobbler's pose with lap baby

Start seated, and bring your feet together, making a diamond shape with your legs. Draw your baby into your lap, so they are facing you, their head resting on your feet. Wrap your hands around baby and your feet, or position your hands to either side of your feet on the floor. Lean forward and make eye contact with your little one as you breathe here.

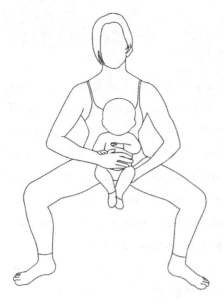

Squat and baby

Start standing with your feet wide, toes slightly pointing out. You might cradle your baby or hold them facing outward or toward your body. Inhale to bend your knees and drop into a squat, and exhale to return to standing. Move between these two shapes several times, allowing your baby to experience the sensation of lifting and lowering. You can play with your stance, taking your feet wider or closer together to change things up for your body.

Down dog with baby stare

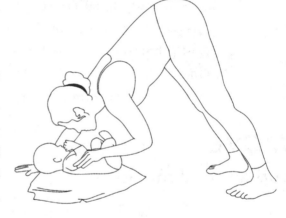

Position your little one resting prone on the ground. You can secure them in blankets or with stuffed animals near them. Come into downward-facing dog so that your head is just above your baby's. As you wiggle, squirm, and explore downward-facing dog, connect with your baby by talking and making faces.

Bridge and baby

Start lying on your back with your knees bent. Depending on the age and abilities of your baby, you could position them lying prone on top of you, belly to belly, or you could sit them up, so that your belly or pelvis is their seat. In either position, make sure you hold on securely to your little one as you lift your hips into bridge pose. You can lift up and down a few times, come into bridge and shimmy your hips, or bring in any other variation you love.

parenting

BREATHE
four-part breath

Sama vritti pranayam is box or equal breathing. This four-part breath involves counting to four on an inhalation, holding for a count of four, exhaling for a count of four, and pausing without breath for a count of four. Because of the focused concentration on counting, and the steady pace and rhythm of this breath practice, box breathing can be helpful in focusing and calming the mind. After all, it's hard to hear the mental chatter when your attention is on counting. This is a simple and effective breath meditation practice for when life seems overwhelming (which, when you're a parent, can feel like most days), and it can be practiced for as many or as few rounds as you would like. As you breathe, aim to inhale and exhale through your nose. If a count of four feels too fast-paced, your box breathing can have a different count, like five or six. The point, though, is to keep all four parts of the breath paced the same, just as all four sides of a square box are the same length.

MOVE
toddler and me yoga

Toddlers are naturally curious, interested, and busy. This practice capitalizes on their natural instincts and brings them to yoga as a source of playful, joyful movement. Keeping toddlers engaged means making noise, singing out the poses, and generally adding in silliness. It's also helpful to keep in mind that this practice may devolve into tickling and playfulness—and that's yoga, too! Erin Hanehan, family and children's yoga teacher, offered us this sweet sequence.

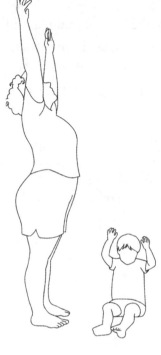

Arms up high and down low

With your toddler, practice lifting your arms "way up high" and moving them "way down low." Ask your child to practice doing this as slowly as they can and then try to mirror each other's movements so that both of you are moving in time and connecting with the other. If they get bored of going slow, try it quicker!

Lift halfway up

Let go of a big breath and fold all the way forward. If you're across from your yoga friend, practice lifting halfway up a few times and giving each other a peek-a-boo look, or a big smile. You can add in silly noises here as you lift up.

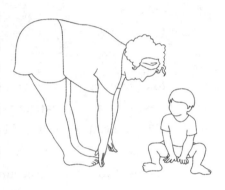

Cobra pose

Get on your bellies and pretend you're snakes slithering around in the grass or the forest. A few times, lift your chest off the ground when you breathe in, just like a cobra. When you breathe out, lie back down on the ground again. Hissing is encouraged!

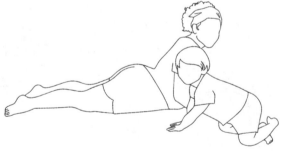

Down dog

From cobra pose, both of you can lift your hips up toward the sky, pretending you're dogs taking a big stretch in the morning. Wiggle your tails and take big breaths in through your nose as though you were sniffing for yummy food. Yipping and barking are allowed.

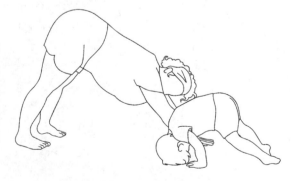

parenting

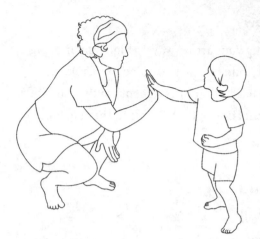

Squatting frog

From down dog, walk forward to the front of your mat and step your feet to the edges of the mat. Squat down between your feet, pretending to transform into a little frog. Your little one might play around with jumping a bit like a little frog.

Star pose

Come up to a standing position and step your feet far away from each other and extend your arms wide to either side. Pretend you are stars in the sky, shining your light out from the center of your belly through your arms, legs, and the tops of your heads. Encourage your little one to stretch out and take up space. You can add loud sighs or another engaging breath here, too.

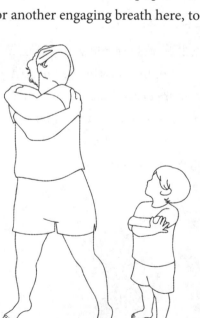

Self-hug

Wrap your arms around yourself and give yourself a big hug, taking several breaths here. (You can also turn this into a joint hug!)

REFLECT
metta meditation

One of our favorite meditation practices comes from Buddhism. In that spiritual tradition, the word *metta* means kindness or goodwill. Metta meditation is also called loving-kindness meditation. The purpose of the practice is to grow your capacity for compassion and empathy, including your capacity for self-empathy. Trust the process of moving toward self-love and connection to others, knowing that self-love, self-empathy, and compassion and empathy for others are exceptional tools for parenting.

To start, get comfortable. Imagine someone that you love with ease: This may be a parent, friend, partner, or child. Visualize them in your mind; imagine details, like the way their hair falls or the crinkles around their eyes. With them in mind, think these lines in your mind, directing the energy of love to them:

May you be safe
May you be healthy
May you be happy
May you live in ease

Next, imagine the larger sense of community you live in: This might be your workplace colleagues, the grocery clerks at your favorite store, the students you often see in yoga class. You can imagine a single person to represent the whole, or you can let these familiar people flicker through your mind for a moment. Then, with your community in mind, direct the energy of love to them, hearing these words again in your mind:

May you be safe
May you be healthy
May you be happy
May you live in ease

parenting

Finally, think of yourself. It may be helpful to imagine a favorite picture you have of yourself or even visualize an image of yourself as a child. Holding yourself in mind, and sending loving-kindness energy to yourself, hear these words:

May I be safe
May I be healthy
May I be happy
May I live in ease

MOVE
family yoga play

Preschoolers and elementary-age children want to do what you're doing. They want to parrot you, be like you, and be with you. This practice is a sweet way to include them and move with them. As with toddler yoga, this practice will likely devolve into silliness and laughter, and that's just fine. You don't need any props, but practicing these in a carpeted space (in case of falls) might be wise.

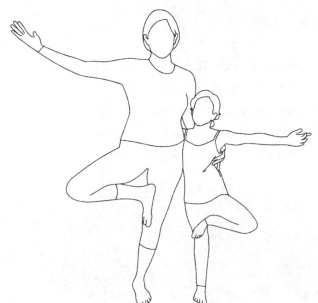

Double tree

Stand with your right leg next to your child's left leg. Place your left foot on the inside of your right leg and have them do the same with their outer leg. Your arms closest to each other can wrap around each other for stability and support while your outer arms reach outward and upward. Try this on one side and then switch sides and try it again.

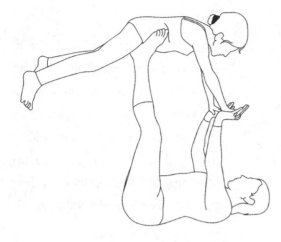

Flying child

Come on to your back with your knees bent and have your child stand near your feet. Bring your feet to their hips and help them find stability by bringing your hands to their shoulders or holding their hands. Count to three together and lift them into the air, "flying" them overhead, balanced on your feet. Practice breathing together and finding calm.

One-legged down dog

You can practice this together or one at a time. From downward-facing dog, you can each extend your right legs toward the ceiling. Once there, you can move your leg around bending it or straightening it or even circling it. See if you can find slow breaths, although if there is laughter or exclamations of "Whoa!" that's okay, too. Rest between sides, and then try this same pose with your left legs extended.

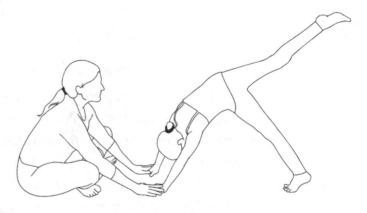

Walking lion

Each of you take downward-facing dog, and then widen your feet until you can comfortably bend your knees. Start to walk your lions around, stepping hands and feet and trying out growls, roars, and lion's breath pranayama.

Parenting

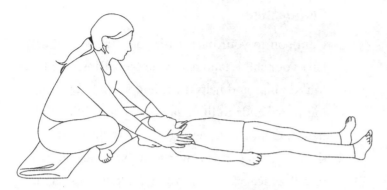

Savasana assists

This pose gives you a chance to offer simple, relaxing touch to your child. Have them come into savasana and close their eyes. You may try rubbing their feet and ankles, giving them a head massage, or sweeping touches lightly over their face. You might try chanting, singing a lullaby, or *OM*ing here, too. (This is Alexandra's daughter's favorite part of family yoga!)

RELATE

Melissa, yogi and mom to a second grader, reflects on the superpower of motherhood.

In Sanskrit, the word for pregnant woman is *dvihṛdayā,* which means two-hearted (*dvi* = two, *hṛdayā* = heart). I love this so much because I think it really encapsulates the vulnerability and bravery that it takes to literally grow a second heart that ultimately lives outside your body without the protection of skin, bones, and muscles. To me, it's a symbol of what it means to be a parent and to engage in the practice of loving your child—regardless of whether or not you physically carried your child or are biologically related to your child. Being a parent and loving your child requires being in close touch with the fragility of life so that you can try to fully appreciate and savor each precious moment, and can also forgive yourself when you don't. It also means loving your child, and yourself, even and especially when it's hard—showing up in some capacity even when you're tired, apologizing after raising your voice, addressing unhelpful patterns and tendencies so that you can model different ones, taking care of yourself even when it disappoints others, giving yourself permission to not be a superhuman, maybe even trying to give your child what you may have missed in your own childhood. It also means finding ways to cultivate happiness in a world full of suffering, without bypassing or denying that suffering, and honoring both when your child is thriving and when they are struggling.

Letting a vulnerable heart live outside your body is a superpower. Loving when it's hard is a superpower. Acknowledging the limits to what you can control and how you can protect your child is a superpower. Allowing your child to make their own mistakes and to experience hurt and rejection, without stepping in to save them, is a superpower. Teaching your child about the injustice and suffering in the world, without sugarcoating it, is a superpower. Navigating life with imperfection, humility, patience, self-sacrifice, compassionately firm boundaries, self-forgiveness, self-reflection, willingness to be wrong, and commitment to change are superpowers. Learning to carry and hold space for it all is a superpower. As parents, we are constantly building our arsenal of never-ending superpowers; sometimes it's fine-tuning old ones, sometimes it's acquiring new ones, and sometimes it's discovering ones we didn't know we had in us or that are more powerful than we ever could have imagined.

WISDOM
your children and the fruits of your actions

In the Hindu epic tale, *The Bhagavad Gita*, the warrior Arjuna has a lengthy discussion with the god Krishna. In the poem, Arjuna confesses some misgivings about the battle he is about to enter, and Krishna's advice is that Arjuna should do his duty with no attachment to the outcome. Krishna says, "Do your duty, but do not concern yourself with the results. We have the right to do our duty, but the results are not dependent only upon our efforts."

This message is a valuable reminder for parenting: We are only responsible for our actions, but not the fruit of our actions. Parenting does not give us full control of our children or their choices. We can offer them love and support, but we can't control the result of that love and support.

parenting

WISDOM
show yourself some grace

We hear a lot about "mom guilt"—the guilt and shame that show up because somehow, despite our best intentions, we perceive ourselves to be failing to love our children in the way we want to or in the way they need. Our student Hannah relayed a moment when she realized mom guilt was endemic and unhelpful:

"During one of our prenatal classes, I remember emotion bubbling up from deep inside when it was my turn to share with the group. It was a time when I felt like I was not a graceful mother—I was pregnant with my second and was not enjoying playing on the floor with my toddler. I felt like I could not be a good mother to my son because I felt so physically taxed. My tears were met with empathy and nods of recognition from others who had felt the same way. After class my teacher told me something that has stuck with me—she shared that she'd had feelings of guilt that her daughter *didn't* have a sibling. She reminded me that 'mom guilt' can creep in, no matter what decisions we make, and that it's a side effect of being a good mother."

When you feel badly about the work you're doing in the role of mother, it hinders you. Sadness and remorse drive guilt, so if you feel badly about some action or situation, reflect on it. But also recognize that over the course of mothering, you won't always be able to rectify every moment of imperfect parenting. There will always be moments where you wish you'd made different choices.

As mothers, sometimes it feels like we are holding the world in a place through a precarious balancing act. A lot falls to us—both in obvious, tangible ways and in vague, less-defined ways. We are constantly remembering details, tending to the fires of relationships, and subtly managing our households. One of our yoga-for-motherhood retreat attendees told us years ago that in the most stressful of times, her mantra is "Choose what to fail." In recognizing that you can't possibly do it all, choosing what to fail sets you up for better success. In any given moment, choosing to fail may mean ordering takeout again, letting the laundry pile up, taking a sick day at work, or canceling plans. Choosing to fail is an act of self-compassion.

Self-compassion is the necessary ability to offer yourself grace, kindness, acceptance, forgiveness, and understanding—just as you would offer it to others. Consider your relationship to your mom-friends. Because mom guilt is so pervasive, it's likely that one of them has confided her perceived failings and the attendant emotional weight to you. In response, did you agree that she was indeed an awful mother who clearly broke off more than she could handle? Or did you reassure her that motherhood is a challenge, and we all feel overwhelmed and ill-prepared for it sometimes? Did you meet her vulnerability by creating a moment of shared humanity? We bet that you did. You can offer that same compassion and empathy to yourself.

baby and me yoga

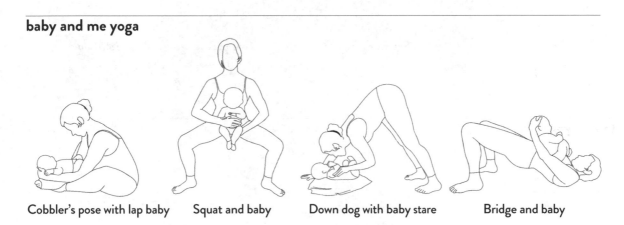

Cobbler's pose with lap baby   Squat and baby   Down dog with baby stare   Bridge and baby

toddler and me yoga

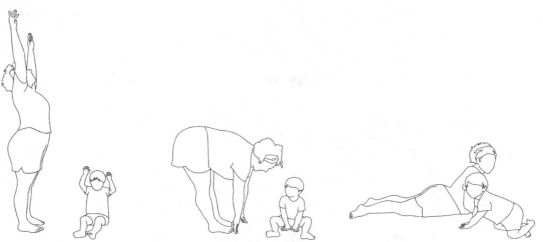

Arms up high and down low   Lift halfway up   Cobra pose

toddler and me yoga (continued)

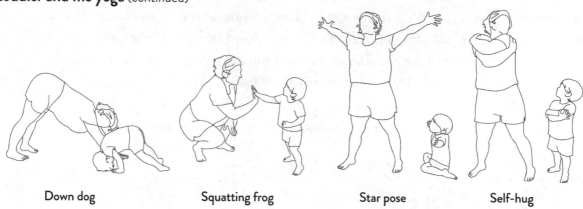

Down dog

Squatting frog

Star pose

Self-hug

family yoga play

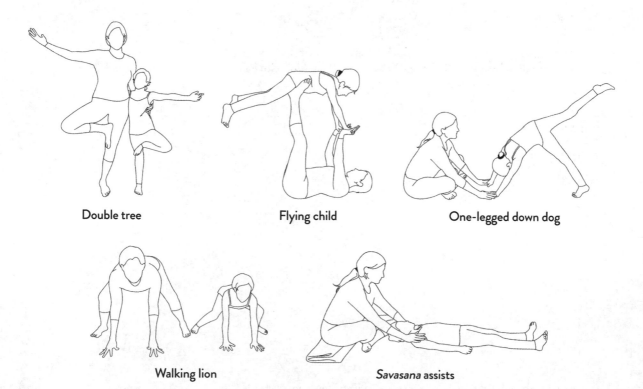

Double tree

Flying child

One-legged down dog

Walking lion

Savasana assists

Chapter Twelve

the family that yogas together . . .

As you change and grow as a mother and parent, so, too, will your yoga practice evolve. Not only are your children growing, changing, and rapidly transitioning to independent creatures, your body might continue its transition from maiden to mother to matriarch to crone. Your hormonal cycle might be shifting and changing; the way you relate to your body and your sexuality might be shifting and changing, too. This is important because *you* are the variable in all your relationships, including the one you have with your children and the one you have with yoga.

With yoga, you get to shift your practice to meet your needs. Yoga is infinitely adaptable, both the asana and pose part of it, and the philosophical messaging of it. It's a spiritual practice that offers you an array of ways to make sense of the world and your life. It's a physical practice that asks you to find shapes that feel good and healing to your body, and when those shapes no longer serve you, you get to leave them behind. Your yoga adapts to your needs, much in the way that you adapt to your children's needs. As they develop and learn to live in the modern world, they need you in different ways: Sometimes they need you to nurture, sometimes set safe boundaries, sometimes they need you to fight their battles, sometimes they need empowerment to fight their own. Always, through

205

parenting

it all, they are watching you for guidance on how to be a human being. No pressure there, right?

We often joke that the early years of parenting are labor intensive (diapers, carrying children, constant snack making), but the later years are *existentially* intensive, as you wrestle more with the "right" way to parent your children, the "right" things to say, the "right" way to love them. It takes a lot of spiritual and emotional work to arrive at your philosophy of parenting—and maybe even more work to implement it in the midst of your daily emotions, shifts, and cycles. If you sometimes feel deeply exhausted or depleted as a result of the hard work of mothering, well, there is a yoga practice that may help with that, too.

It takes a lot of spiritual and emotional work to arrive at your philosophy of parenting.

In yoga philosophy, the *kleshas* are the obstacles to enlightenment or the causes of suffering. The Sanskrit word *klesha* means "poison" or "affliction," and indeed, one way of thinking about the kleshas is that each one is a spiritual affliction we must grapple with. The first two kleshas can offer us helpful tools to guide our parenting approach.

The first klesha is *avidya*, which means "wrong seeing" or ignorance. When we see things incorrectly, we obviously don't respond in ways that align with our deeper intentions—or act in correct ways, either. So much of connecting with your child is about communication: making sure you talk so that they can hear you and understand you and also listening so that they feel heard and understood. To move from avidya to *vidya* (seeing clearly), you have to consider perspectives other than your own. That may mean listening deeper to your child or consulting your partner, a trusted mom friend, or a parenting expert. Part of yoga is cultivating a stronger relationship with yourself so that the loudest voice you hear is your own. But that doesn't mean you shouldn't seek out perspectives from therapists or loved ones. Expanding your knowledge and your view can mean that you suddenly see much more clearly.

The second klesha is *asmita*, most often translated to mean "ego." We often joke that there's no dignity in parenting (we're thinking here of the many times our children have interrupted us in the bathroom, for instance), but despite that lack of dignity, ego remains. In our limited experience, ego shows up more as our children get older and start to do what's incredibly healthy and normal: challenge us. Ego is what kicks in and thinks, *I'm right* or *I'm in charge.* And while drawing healthy boundaries is essential for creating a sense of safety for our children, when ego is at the root of those boundaries, they become dividers, not keeping our children safe, but separating them from our love. Ego is self-righteous. Ego is sensitive and insecure. Ego is easily angered. The way we move past ego's hold on us is to be vulnerable with our children. One of our favorite reminders for our children is this: "I was never a parent before you. I'm learning on the job." It's a humble reminder for both them and us that we are bound to make mistakes along the way. Expressing this vulnerability pushes ego to the side; it lessens the division between our children and ourselves.

No one approach to parenting is the right approach because there are so many variables. And your approach will shift as time passes and they grow, and you *also* continue to change.

MOVE
yoga for when you're angry

Anger is an emotion that feels especially challenging to navigate. It may feel out of place in the context of yoga, but anger happens, and it often happens for very good reasons—truly, how long does it take the kids to find their shoes? Could someone else (*anyone* else?) start the laundry? The frustrations of everyday parenting can build and build. Sometimes we feel anger in a healthy way—there are a lot of injustices around motherhood, including a lack of maternal leave and support in America. But sometimes our anger is driven by fear or ego—our children reject us, our ideas, or our sense of what is right. In those instances, the experience of anger or how we express it can make us feel out of control, disconnected from ourselves, and unaligned with our truest intentions. Anger is a common emotion for new parents to experience, as everything is changing so rapidly and the parenting responsibilities seem endless—and it's a common emotion for all parents to feel because, truly, the parenting responsibilities *are* endless. When you feel mad—at the laundry or lost shoes or lack of maternal support or any number of real and true things—try this practice:

parenting

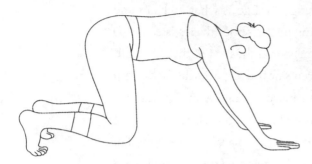

Down dog with knee tucks

Start in downward-facing dog. As you inhale, bend your knees and drop your weight further into your feet. As you exhale, spring back into downward-facing dog. You may sigh out of your mouth on the exhale. Repeat this until it feels fatiguing.

Standing goddess twists

Come to the top of your mat, and step your feet, toes pointed outward, as wide as your mat or wider. Drop into a squat where your pelvis and thighs are about parallel to one another. Place your hands on your thighs and lock your arms, so that the weight of your upper body is supported by your hands. Allow your chest to drop forward and toward the ground. Inhale, and as you exhale, twist from your belly, drawing one shoulder forward. Repeat this to the other side, inhaling through the center and exhaling to drop the opposite shoulder forward.

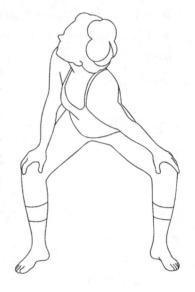

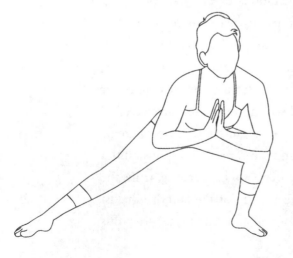

Flowing squat

Face the long edge of your mat, and step your feet wide apart. Bring your hands to your heart. Inhale, and as you exhale, shift your weight to your left leg, bending your left knee, so you are in a half-squat. Inhale as you move your torso through the midline. As you exhale, shift your weight to your right leg, bending your right knee. Continue to shift side to side for several breaths.

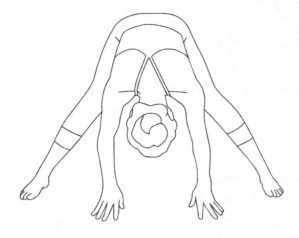

Wide-legged forward fold hang

Step your feet as wide as feels pleasant to you, with your feet parallel to each other. Inhale to sweep your arms overhead, and as you exhale, fold forward, coming into a wide-legged forward fold. In this shape, you can hang and allow gravity to traction your spine. You can also sway, sweep your hands behind your back, or walk your hands forward or backward of your body. Your legs can stay fully straight, or you can explore bending one knee at a time. Take your time in this shape.

Puppy pose

Come to hands and knees and walk your hands forward and wider than your mat. Lower your head toward the floor, allowing your forehead to touch

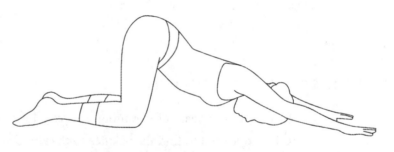

down. Your hips should stay aligned over your knees. You can lower your elbows to the floor or keep your arms taut and extended. As you inhale, feel your heart melt downward, and as you exhale feel a slight lift upward in your body.

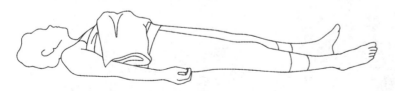

Blanket hug *savasana*

Take a blanket and fold it longways several times, until it resembles a long, rectangular snake. Wrap this blanket around your body, along your bra line, and wrap the ends one on top of the other across your chest. Lie down and take savasana with the blanket "hugging" you and offering your rib cage gentle lift. Rest here.

parenting

BREATHE
the three-breath hug

This breath practice is a family practice! Our families use this to help connect with one another, find calm, and bring attention back to our bodies. We call this breath a three-breath hug, but in reality, once you're in it, you might decide to stay for longer. To practice with your family, set up for a big hug—you might explain to your partner or child the purpose of the breath hug, so they can bring awareness and mindfulness into the practice, too. Take a moment to stand still and slow your breathing. Notice the pressure of your body against your child's or partner's. See if you can sync your breath and take in a joint inhale, releasing your exhale at the same pace and rhythm. Practice this for three rounds of breath (or longer) and notice how it shifts your energy, increasing sense of connection to your loved one.

MOVE
yoga for space and self-care

Since the later years of parenting involve a lot more existential and psychological work, it's important to find the balance to that in time alone, space, and self-care. This spacious practice offers some pleasant hip opening and gives you a chance to check in with your shoulders, upper back, and deeper self, too. Sometimes we need silence and space to make the leap from avidya to vidya. The cherry on top in this sweet practice is the extra cozy savasana—give yourself ample time to experience and enjoy that grand finale pose that offers an important chunk of self-care time. For this sequence, you'll want all the props.

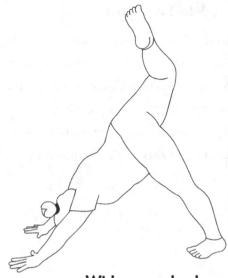

Down dog with hip circles

Come into downward-facing dog and extend your right leg high into the air. Keep your shoulders level and stack your right hip on top of your left hip as you bend your right knee, allowing your right foot to drop over to the left. Make small circles with your knee. The size of the circles you are making with your right knee may remain small, or you might increase the size. At some point, reverse the direction of the movement of your circles. Repeat this dynamic pose on the left side.

Wide-armed cobra play

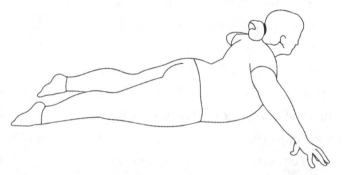

From down dog, shift forward into plank and then lower down to your belly. Bring your arms a little wider than shoulder distance apart and slightly in front of your mat. Rise up onto your fingertips, lifting up through your chest and creating space across the front of your body. Take turns dipping your left shoulder toward the ground, gazing right, and then dipping your right shoulder toward the ground, gazing left. Move through this two or three times.

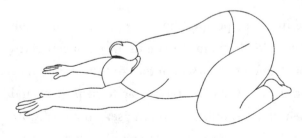

Child's pose

From cobra, press into your hands and lift your seat to come up to a tabletop position. Bring your big toes together and separate your knees as far as is comfortable before bringing your hips back to rest on your heels for child's pose. You might play around with extending your arms long in front of you and walking your hands over to one side of the mat and then the other.

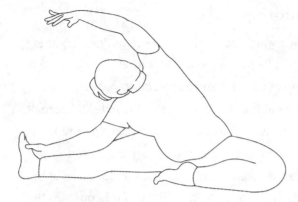

Revolved head-to-knee pose

Have a seat on the floor and draw your left foot in toward your inner right thigh. Keep space in your right side body and extend your right arm down the length of your right leg. Stretch your left arm up and alongside your ear, drawing your shoulder blade onto your back. Repeat this on the second side.

All-the-props *savasana*

Gather your bolster, two blocks, wash-cloth, or eye pillow, and three blankets. Place your blocks at the lowest, or second lowest height, in a T-position at the back

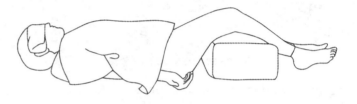

of your mat. Place your bolster under your knees. Fold two blankets such that, when you lie down, you are able to place the blankets under your arms to support them. You can place your third blanket on top of you or fold it further and place it over your belly or hips. Place your washcloth or eye pillow over your eyes to make this extra sweet.

REFLECT
rooted like a tree

One of our favorite chants came from our postpartum student, Ruth. The main phrase of it—rooted like a tree—makes a wonderful mantra on its own. But combined with the other lines, it can be sung or chanted to yourself, in the context of your yoga practice, or (how we have often used it) to our children as a way to help them find their own sense of groundedness when they feel unbalanced or upset emotionally. It's a reminder for your children (and you!) that emotions are the weather, but they are the stable, rooted tree. This chant has been especially important for Alexandra and her daughter, now seven. When her daughter feels dysregulated, afraid, or overwhelmed, she often asks to be "rooted," and they chant this chant together.

Rooted like a tree
I am rooted like a tree
Roots grow so deep
I am rooted like a tree
Everything will change
Nothing stays the same
And through it all
My roots will remain

MOVE
yoga for physical imbalance

We don't know if one side always felt quite different from the other, but aging, birth, and motherhood definitely seem to have made it more obvious, right? As your children grow older and you can tune back into your body more, you may notice little differences that weren't as obvious when you were completely immersed in mothering. If you have one side of your torso, one hip, or one leg that feels a little less awake and turned on, this is an excellent sequence for you. As you practice it, you can give equal attention to both sides, or you can focus on holding longer on the side that feels like it needs more time. One block and use of a wall will be helpful here.

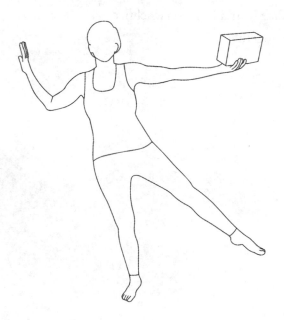

One-legged lift at the wall

Stand parallel to a wall and put your closest arm against it. Place your block in your outside hand. As you inhale, lift both your hand with the block and the leg beneath it. Do this lift several times, until you feel a sense of effort in your legs.

Side body stretch at the wall

From this same pose, sweep your outside arm overhead, so that your block touches the wall just above or behind your head. At the same time, send your lifted leg behind you, and bend your front knee, as if you were doing a curtsy.

Play between these first two poses, inhaling to lift your leg and arm out, and exhaling to settle your block against the wall and find the curtsy. Repeat these poses and explorations on the second side.

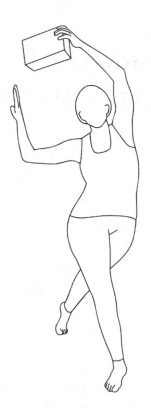

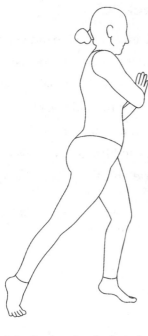

Single leg calf raise with kickstand

In standing, bring your hands to your heart and slide your right foot behind you, propping onto the ball of that foot or even just your toes. Think of your right foot as a kickstand; there is some weight on it, but it's just there for balance support. Inhale as you rise up to the ball of your left foot and exhale as you lower your left heel back down. Repeat this ten to twenty times. If this starts to feel easy and you want more challenge, try this without the kickstand, described below.

Balancing single leg calf raise

In standing, bring your hands to your heart and bend your left leg to lift your left calf and foot behind you. From a controlled place of balance, inhale to rise to the ball of your right foot and exhale to lower that foot back down. If it feels impossible to lower with a sense of control, skip these for now and focus on the iteration of this pose described previously.

Repeat single leg calf raises on the second side.

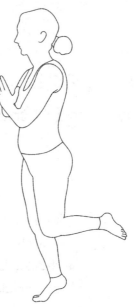

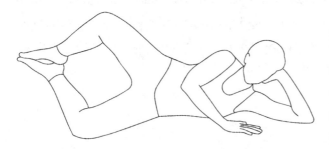

Side-lying clam

Come to lie on your side on your mat. Prop your head on your hand, resting your elbow and upper arm on the floor. Your top hand can rest on the floor in front of your chest. Bend your knees, and imagine you are gluing the big-toe sides of your feet together. Tip your knees toward the ground and lift your feet into the air. Inhale. As you exhale, pull your top knee away from your bottom knee, making a diamond shape with your legs. This is a movement, so inhale to close your knees back together and exhale to open them again. Continue this until your top outer hip feels appropriately fatigued, and then set up to repeat this movement on the second side.

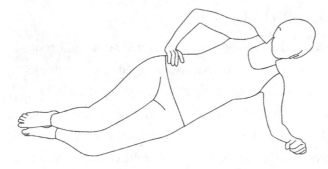

Supported side plank

From this same side lying position, bend your knees and come to your forearm. Your top hand can rest on your hip. Inhale. As you exhale, push the floor away and come into a side plank. You can practice this as a movement a few times (inhale to lower, exhale to lift), and then eventually come into the side plank and stay there for several breaths.

Repeat this pose on the second side.

REFLECT
savoring (?) the chaos

Savoring every moment of your child's childhood is an impossibility. Just like you can't find absolute balance between the sides of your body, you can't be fully present for every aspect of your child's life. Please know this when a well-meaning older man or woman gazes into your very soul and tells you to "Enjoy every moment. It goes so fast." Time has a way of doing that, no matter how much you "savor" it or let it pass, mind in the clouds. Practicing mindfulness and developing a yoga and meditation practice can be helpful, though, in developing more present-moment awareness, something that has been shown to seemingly slow time down (in a good way).

MOVE
yoga for feeling overwhelmed

Feeling exhausted physically, feeling overwhelmed by emotions (or a sense of "How do I handle *this*?") is part of the motherhood and parenthood experience. When children are little, the questions and answers are often exhausting, but simple: "Can you help me tie my shoes?" But as children age, parenting requires so much more emotional bandwidth as the questions become increasingly complex, and the answers aren't always clear: "Can I spend the night at my friend's house?" "Why do I need to go to school?" "Why do you get to make all the rules?" Lauren's tween son told her yesterday that he "had never been so stressed in his life." (He's currently in the school play.) It's hard to help children deal with their emotions when we feel overwhelmed by our own. This little sequence moves you through poses that give you a chance to say hello to your spine, hips, and body—even when you're feeling as though you don't have all (or any!) of the answers.

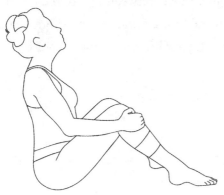

Seated cow

Start seated with your knees bent and your feet planted in front of you, hip distance apart. Grasp your legs: either your shins or the backs of your thighs. As you inhale, use your arms to help you pull your body forward, lifting your heart.

Seated cat

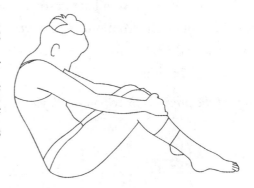

From the same position, start to exhale, and round your spine, leaning back and letting your body receive some traction from the grasp of your arms on your legs. Move between seated cow and cat for as many breaths as feels good.

Side-sitting heart-opening

From the same seated position, start to drop your knees side to side. Enjoy the glutes massage that comes from that movement. Finally, allow your knees to drop to the right. Take a moment to adjust your body: Your knees might stack or slide away from each other. You might move your right hand farther from your body, so your hand and shoulder

parenting

are at a wider angle from each other. (You can even come down to your right forearm, if you'd like.) With an inhale, reach your left arm up and back, feeling your heart-space open.

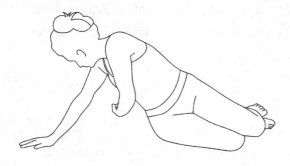

Side-sitting thread through

From this same position, begin your exhale, and sweep your left arm through space. Reach your left arm under your body as if you were threading it under you. Round your spine. Move between this pose and the previous one several times. Inhale to open your heart and exhale to reach your lifted arm under your body.

Side-sitting thread through pause

Eventually, as you thread your left arm under your body, pause and draw your left forearm to the mat and then your right. Continue to allow your heart and torso to drift away from your knees. Rest here for as many breaths as you'd like.

Repeat the previous three poses with your knees to the left.

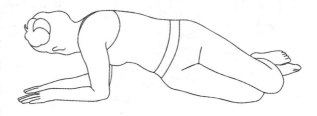

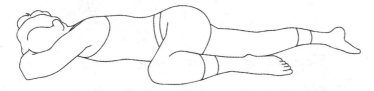

Prone half frog

For this last pose, roll onto your belly and use your hands under your head as a pillow. You can rest your forehead on your hands or turn your head in whatever direction feels most natural. Slide your right knee up and out, as if you were making a tree pose shape, but on your belly. (Your right foot does not need to touch your left leg; it can be tucked in toward your body or even shifted out from it.) Rest here and breathe, finding the sweet spot between settling in and making an effort.

Repeat this pose with your left knee out to the side.

RELATE
the transformative power of yoga on mothering

Sommer Sobin, cofounder of Thousand Petals Yoga and mom to an elementary-age child and middle schooler, on how her yoga practice is integral to her parenting.

Yoga has been my most treasured resource. It gives me a place to replenish, to embrace the necessary friction of growth, and it opens my heart so I am able to parent with love, compassion, and forgiveness.

Meeting life as it is (the practice of welcoming in the divine mess) has been one of my greatest teachers. As an introvert drawn toward silence and simplicity, parenting has challenged me and pushed me to develop new skills and to find creative ways to make sure my inner needs are met. I've had to let go of control mechanisms, let go of false perfectionism as the laundry piled up, learn to go with the unexpected scheduling changes when suddenly a child is home sick for the day, and learn how to laugh more while cherishing and riding the waves. My mat is always unrolled in the middle of my living room, beckoning me, even if for just a few spare moments, as it's my place of refuge. Some days I drag myself there, some days I count the seconds until I get to practice, and some days I just sit for a few minutes in stillness, even as the noise of the household envelops my attempts at peace and quiet.

More recently, my practice has shifted to a place of ceremony. After twelve-plus years of parenting, and struggling to find consistent practice time since then, I finally went against my long-held narrative that I was not a morning person. I have now embraced a 5:30 AM practice time as my daily holy time. The alarm goes off and regardless of my initial thoughts, I roll out of bed and step onto my mat for thirty to forty-five minutes. The practice of feeling my body, not being swayed by my mind's preferences, and the willingness to move through grief, sadness, yesterday's worries, and to center myself with love in all that I do has been the most transformative commitment I've made in over twenty-five years of practice. I find that when I tend to myself in this way, I feel alive in my body, my inner realms feel tended to, and I am a more compassionate and available parent. I'm also able to pause more and course correct on the days when my fuse runs short. The inner static is quieter, and I can listen to my children's needs more clearly because I've done the same for myself.

parenting

WISDOM

abhinivesha: all our fears as mothers

Alexandra talks about the looming fear that is central for so many mothers.

I worry about my daughter dying more often than I can even bear to write out. I know that you, too, fear for your children's lives because it's part of the package of motherhood—the scariest, darkest fears cross our minds. With motherhood, we've arrived at a place where there is so much to lose. Too much to lose. Too much of a loss to even comprehend. Even writing about this makes my stomach hurt—it makes this always-back-there-fear rise into my throat, where no amount of gulping will send it away.

The fear begins when we're pregnant. We pray and hope our way through that first trimester, when even the least interested-in-pregnancy among us know that there is a greater chance of miscarriage. Moments of fear come and go through pregnancy and for some of us, they crescendo in the chaos of birth—the unknown experience that can feel both natural and foreign. And then our babes are born, and a new fear arises, a clear and persistent fear: We must keep them alive.

In fact, the first few months of motherhood is silently punctuated by the phrase "please thrive." So much of the anxiety of the first days, weeks, and months is about this fragile, soft, tiny being who you alone are now fully responsible for keeping safe and sound. Looking back, I can see how that was always in the background of my first year with my daughter, but I never spoke about it then. How could I even put that terror into words when she was so delicate, so freshly created? How can any new mother find those words?

I don't think my thoughts about this are pathological, although I admit that the shadow of this fear crosses my mind regularly. I think these anxieties are in line with what it means to have children—especially in this day and age when we get so much information about just how much there is to fear. A cursory scroll through any mothers' group on social media will quickly remind you that strangers, expired car seats, and even cookie dough are all out to get our children. People have expressed this persistent, low-level distress in many ways: Our babies are our hearts walking around outside our bodies—that's a good way to say it. Francis Bacon said, "He that hath . . . children, hath given hostages to fortune." I quite like that one: When we bring our babies into this world and love them in this crazy deep way, we are putting our lives, their lives, our sanity into the hands of fate—and never have the odds felt so scary and precarious, simply because there are odds at all.

One helpful thing to remember is that technology, medicine, and modern society are on our side, even if the messaging we get via social media is not. Despite fears and anxieties, data shows that our children have never been safer; looking at rates of death for children under five from 1800 to the present day reveals that the outlook is good for your child thriving and surviving, especially when compared against the past. According to statistics from the World Health Organization, mortality rates for children under the age of five have decreased by nearly 60% since the late 1990s. That's pretty calming, if you ask me. (But it's not enough, of course, because nothing could ever be enough except a 100 percent guarantee of a lifetime of happiness, safety, and health.)

So, what do we do about this fear—this fear that is the main anxiety of motherhood?

In yoga, the kleshas are seen as the causes of suffering that we must wrestle with in order to find a life of ease. The last klesha is *abhinivesha*. Abhinivesha is the fear of death or attachment to life. Abhinivesha is seen as the pinnacle obstacle to happiness—in order to be truly at peace, yoga philosophy suggests we have to confront our fear of death. Maybe it sheds light on how the ancient history of yoga is mostly meditative, ascetic men doing the practice because there is not a klesha that means "fear of loss of children." Like all moms everywhere, my own life matters less than that of my child. Still, the fear we have for our children's lives is abhinivesha, too.

To move through this fear and begin to see it clearly, the starting point is acknowledgment and acceptance.

Here is the truth: One day, you are going to die. And one day, so is your child.

Deep breath in.

Deep breath out.

One of my favorite takes on death acceptance comes from a comedy bit called "Happy Endings" that Stephen Colbert did on one of his shows. In it, he discusses research that suggests when people know the ending of a story, they enjoy the story more. From that, he surmises that we all know the ending of our own story. The punch line is: You die. But, he says, doesn't knowing this—accepting that that is indeed the definite end of your story—help you enjoy the story more?

Ram Dass says, "Being here now is experiential. When you are in the moment, time slows down. In this moment you have all the time in the world. *But don't waste a moment.*" Existential psychology posits that facing death fear and anxiety brings positive benefits. When people are surrounded by reminders of death, they tend to embrace a desire to live life more authentically.

If I remember that one day my daughter will die (and so will I) and if I allow my anxiety of this fear to become an emblem of the sweetness of this short and fleeting life, well then, can't that fear be transformed into a poignant reminder to live fully? When I feel that fear in my throat, when that shadow crosses into my thoughts, can't it become a prompt that connects me to authentically living—being in the moment and savoring the gift of my child's life in the face of understanding that the end will come, and I have no control of when that may be?

I think so. I hope so. That's what I'm working on, anyway.

WISDOM
mother is a verb

Our friend and yoga colleague Anna Jefferson wrote this poem about motherhood and shared it in a yoga for motherhood group.

Mother is a verb. She is composed of action.
Like carry. Like bleed. Protect.
To mother is to respond: to listen. Play. Cuddle. Observe. Wash. Remind. Plan— but also improvise.

Mother is a verb like hold: little hands and little bodies, special sticks, discarded jackets. Holding court, holding your secrets, holding you in her heart. Holding all of this together; she is holding on.

Mother is a verb that, in its repetition, alchemically transmutes her verb into a noun.

Labor

Diaper

Bandage

Nurse

Cook

Hug

Nag

Balance

Kiss

She is answers, she is questions.

Has she become a thing? Somehow her action rendered still, like a statue—the sweaty acts of her creation become inert, invisible.

Mother is an hourglass,

a solid thing composed of tiny movements through time.

But as Krishna taught Arjuna, she is not entitled

to the fruits of her actions, only to her own ceaseless pulse:

Cultivating

Mentoring

Hoping

And releasing

WISDOM
being a yoga mom

Perhaps one of the most important aspects of yoga as a practice adjacent to parenting is that it is infinitely adaptable. We discuss this at various points in the book, and we see how it's true in our daily lives. Sometimes we practice yoga asana. For both of us, we have had stretches where we've stepped away from the poses and embraced running, weight-training, and other movement classes. We have also recognized times when our bodies have required slower practices—walking in the woods, short summer swims, and meditation before a nap. Regardless of the movement, we

parenting

carry with us the breathwork, intention, and presence that we learned from yoga. In this way, all movement practices are yoga, in that they are all rooted in helping us connect more deeply to ourselves. The philosophies of yoga are guideposts of our mothering. We live in households that om and chant, practice yoga poses, and use breathwork and mindfulness as stress interventions. We are better mothers not just because we practice physical asana, but because we know that yoga's tools help us stay grounded and present. When we come from a place of internal connection, it is that much easier to remain connected and patient with our children. Yoga is so helpful through pregnancy, but it continues to help through the postpartum stage and then through parenting children of all ages.

yoga for when you're angry

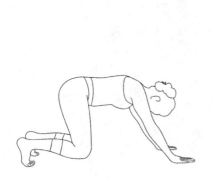

Down dog with knee tucks

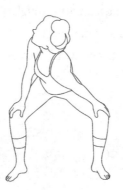

Standing goddess twists

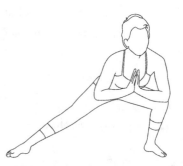

Flowing squat

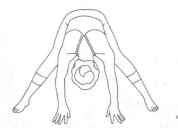

Wide-legged forward fold hang

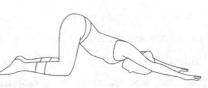

Puppy pose

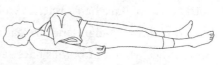

Blanket hug savasana

yoga for space and self-care

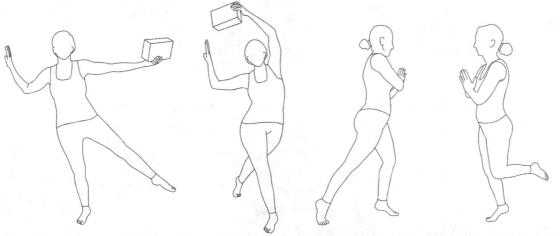

Down dog with hip circles   Wide-armed cobra play   Child's pose

Revolved head-to-knee pose   All-the-props savasana

yoga for physical imbalance

One-legged lift at the wall   Side body stretch at the wall   Single leg calf raise with kickstand   Balancing single leg calf raise

yoga for physical imbalance (continued)

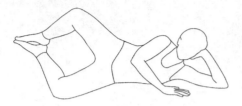

Side-lying clam

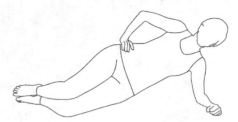

Supported side plank

yoga for feeling overwhelmed

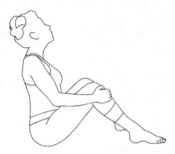

Seated cow

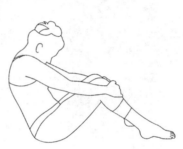

Seated cat

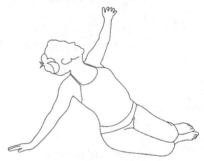

Side-sitting heart-opening

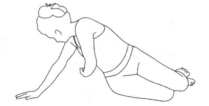

Side-sitting thread through

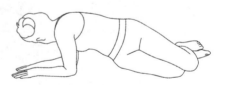

Side-sitting thread through pause

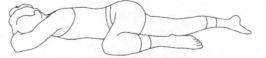

Prone half frog

acknowledgments

Without the insight, compassion, and support of our yoga mentors, our yoga community, colleagues, and students, and our friends and collaborators in perinatal fields, this book would never have been written. Their collective experiences and observations about yoga and motherhood and parenthood are such an important part of this text. We knew we wanted their voices and wisdom here, and we're so grateful that they wrote their thoughts, talked with us, and shared generously so that our readers could bask in their sagacity, too.

We are deeply grateful to Linda Konner, our agent, and Darcie Abbene, our editor at HCI Books, and Larissa Henoch, HCI Art Director for their support and discernment. Our ideas shine brighter because of their help.

Finally, we would not be mothers without our partners and children, whose stories fill these pages, and whose love fills our lives. Thank you especially to these dearest ones.

about the authors

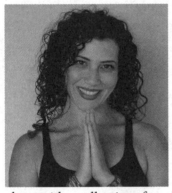

Alexandra DeSiato, MA, E-RYT 500, is an expert in yoga for the prenatal and postpartum time periods. She is recognized internationally for her work on creating (and helping others create) powerful and resonant themes in yoga classes. Her workshops have been offered nationally, including at Yogaville Ashram in Virginia and Kripalu Yoga and Healing Arts Center in the Berkshires of Massachusetts. Together with Lauren, she cofounded and coleads Whole Mama Yoga (wholemamayoga.com), where they, along with a collective of teachers, offer fertility, prenatal, postpartum, and motherhood yoga classes. Alexandra and Lauren also coteach a highly lauded prenatal and postpartum yoga teacher training and lead mothering and parenting retreats. Alexandra has co-authored two books with Sage Rountree, *Lifelong Yoga* and *Teaching Yoga Beyond the Poses*. Alexandra holds a master's degree in English literature and, in addition to teaching yoga classes, has taught college writing and literature for more than twenty years. She lives in the Chapel Hill, North Carolina, area with her husband and daughter.

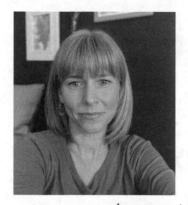

Lauren Sacks, E-RYT 500, PRYT, is a perinatal and hatha yoga instructor with more than twenty years of teaching experience. She was a founding member of Carrboro Yoga Company in 2004 and taught thousands of students during her fifteen-year tenure. Practical alignment, whimsical humor, and fierce authenticity are hallmarks of Lauren's classes. For twelve years, Lauren worked as an event and retreat planner in the field of arts and higher education administration, and draws from her experience there to facilitate retreats that are heart nourishing, soulful, and fun, and expand on the community created through her yoga classes. With Alexandra, Lauren cofounded Whole Mama Yoga (wholemamayoga.com). Along with a collective of teachers, they lead yoga classes, workshops, and other events to support all aspects of parenting—from preconception to perimenopause. Several times a year, Alexandra and Lauren also coteach an internationally renowned Pre and Postnatal Yoga Teacher Training program. Lauren's expertise in perinatal yoga as well as her beloved Yoga for Motherhood classes make her a sought-after presenter in yoga teacher training programs, and she works regularly with both UNC and Duke to teach tools of yoga to residents, obstetricians, midwives, and their patients. Lauren loves reading, cooking, eating, quilting, napping, and her family and friends (in no particular order). She lives in Carrboro, North Carolina, with her husband and their two children.

about the artist

Vivian Iris Rountree (vivianrountree.com) is currently a student at the University of California, Davis, pursuing interests in anthropology and psychology. She creates digital art based on life-forms from humans to animals. She has also produced macrophotography of the interplay of light and water droplets on natural flora.